THE DOCTOR WHO WAS
FOLLOWED BY GHOSTS

THE DOCTOR WHO WAS FOLLOWED BY GHOSTS

a memoir

Dr. Li Qunying and Louis Han

ECW PRESS

Published by ECW PRESS
2120 Queen Street East, Suite 200, Toronto, Ontario, Canada M4E 1E2

LIBRARY AND ARCHIVES CANADA CATALOGUING IN PUBLICATION

Qunying, Li, 1926–
The doctor who was followed by ghosts: the family saga of a
Chinese woman doctor / Li Qunying and Louis Han

ISBN 978-1-55022-781-9

1. Qunying, Li, 1926–. 2. China — History — 20th century.
3. Women physicians — China — Biography. 4. Physicians — China — Biography I.
Han, Louis II. Title.

R604.Q85A3 2007   610.69'5092   C2007-903575-2

Cover, photo gallery and text design: Tania Craan
Typesetting: Mary Bowness
Production: Rachel Brooks
Printed by Friesens

The publication of *The Doctor Who Was Followed by Ghosts* has been
generously supported by the Canada Council for the Arts, which this year
invested $20.1 million in writing and publishing throughout Canada, by the Ontario
Arts Council, by the Government of Ontario through the Ontario Book Publishing Tax
Credit, and the Government of Canada through the Book Publishing Industry
Development Program (BPIDP).

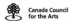 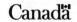 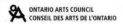

This book is set in Fairfield.

DISTRIBUTION

CANADA: Jaguar Book Group, 100 Armstrong Avenue, Georgetown, ON, L7G 5S4
UNITED STATES: Independent Publishers Group, 814 North Franklin Street,
Chicago, Illinois 60610

PRINTED AND BOUND IN CANADA

ECW PRESS
ecwpress.com

Dedicated to our family.

When his favorite daughter falls ill, Yanwang, the ruler of the underworld, sends his servants to look for a doctor who has as few ghosts as possible following him. This means that he is a better doctor than others, because when a patient dies, its ghost follows and haunts the doctor.

— Chinese folklore

Table of Contents

FOREWORD *xi*

PART I

1. The Fate of a Nun 3

2. Rat—the First Sign of the Horoscope *13*

3. The Eighth Route Army 27

4. The Doctor 37

5. Love and War 47

6. "Valiantly and Spiritedly, I Fell into the Yalu River" 55

7. A Bag of Gold 73

8. The 38th Parallel and the Wedding 85

PART II

9. Peace 93

10. Tiger's Teeth *107*

11. THE YEAR OF THE RAT (1960) *123*

12. "WHERE ARE YOU, DR. LI?" *135*

13. SEEING CHAIRMAN MAO *145*

14. CUTTING PONYTAILS *157*

15. SEPARATION *169*

16. THE INNERMOST SOUL *187*

PART III

17. THE BAREFOOT DOCTOR *207*

18. GOING TO BEIJING *223*

19. REHABILITATION *237*

20. SEEING CHAIRMAN MAO AGAIN *247*

21. EVIL GHOST *261*

AFTERWORD *267*

ABOUT THE AUTHORS *279*

ACKNOWLEDGEMENTS *281*

FOREWORD

———

THIS IS THE STORY of my ill-fated life and struggles through the Anti-Japanese War, Civil War, Korean War, the famine of the early sixties and numerous political movements, including the notorious Cultural Revolution. The Great Leap Forward took away my son Bingbing's life, and the Cultural Revolution took a heavy toll on my husband Han Wende's health, and consequently led to his death before the age of sixty. Besides our personal misfortunes, I also witnessed the suffering of the peasants, who were the majority of the population at the grassroots level and whose stories have rarely been told.

Traumatic twentieth-century China was marked by chaos, war, famine, and oppression. At the dawn of the century, the Chinese empire was decaying, carved up mercilessly by the powerful foreign nations trying to exert as much control over it as possible. In 1900, the anti-foreign Boxer Rebellion broke out as rebels attempted to rid China of Western influences. In 1912, Sun Yat-sen, founder of modern China, overthrew the corrupted Qing Dynasty and established the Republic, which was followed by a period of warlords, leaving China politically fragmented. Warfare marked the first half of the century. Most notable was the protracted Sino-Japanese War as well as the Civil War between the Nationalists and the Communists, following Japan's surrender.

The second half of the century, which began with military involvement in the Korean War, was characterized by frequent and brutal political campaigns including the great famine in the early 1960s under Mao's Communist reign. The struggle to become a modern nation followed — under the rule of Deng Xiaoping, who is remembered as a daring political and economic reformer, and, at the same time, for his bloody military crackdown of the June Fourth student demonstration in 1989, as well as forced abortion and infanticides due to his unpopular "one child policy."

When it comes to impact on the global economy, China is one of the most talked about countries today. However, the peasants are left behind by this seemingly booming economy and still can't afford to see doctors. Epidemic corruption has spread through every level of society, from government officials who claim to be selfless "public servants of the people" to doctors who practice "humanitarianism." Many doctors become corrupt, receiving extravagant commissions from prescribing unnecessary drugs or demanding gifts from patients. Fake medicine produced by people bent solely on profit is prevalent and threatens public health.

My experience is part of a turbulent period in history. Sometimes painful, my story brings together history as I witnessed it, along with folklore and superstition — revealing the brutality, intrigue, and occasional absurdity of life in twentieth-century China.

This memoir is an unfulfilled wish of my deceased husband, Wende. A few years before he passed away, he had — on several occasions — talked about his intention to write the family story. However, his lingering fear of the previous political movements prevented him from doing so.

Two years after Wende passed away, striving to carry out his aspiration, I started writing a family memoir. I completed over fifty pages, from the time I was young through to the Cultural Revolution. But in the end, just like my husband, I became afraid of causing trouble. I burned the writing to ashes.

I am grateful to my youngest son, Luping, and his wife Patty, without whom this book would not have been possible. In 1999, fifteen years after my husband had passed away, Luping (Louis), who lives in Canada, expressed the idea of compiling the memoir. I thought to myself that it might be time to share the story with the rest of the world.

To refresh my memory, I carefully went though all the old letters and scrutinized the time-worn black and white photos that revealed so many stories. Many events were unbearable for me to recall. Among the papers that I had saved was a bundle of letters my husband had written over the years, after being purged during the Cultural Revolution. These letters included copies of appeals made to the army, in which he had once been an officer. I, too, presented his case to the army many times and to the central government in Beijing without achieving any results.

After seven years of hard work, our family story takes on the shape it has now.

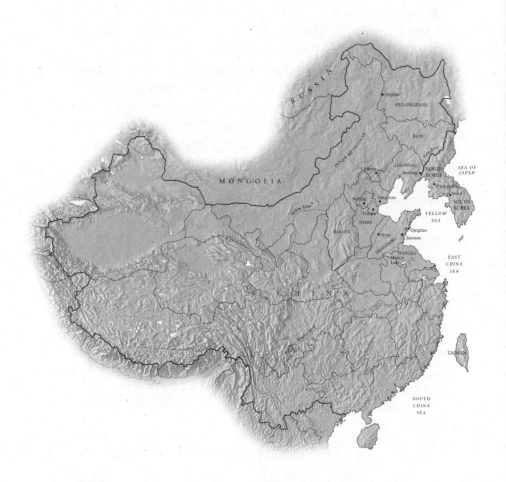

PART I

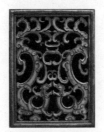

The Fate of a Nun

A MONTH BEFORE MY ninth birthday, my mother took me to a blind fortune-teller in the street. It was a bitterly cold morning in lunar November 1934, a year after the Japanese began to occupy Chifeng City, Inner Mongolia. The fortune-teller touched my face with his coarse hands and revealed my fate.

"Your daughter should never get married," he said.

"What?" My mother was shaken by the bleak prediction. She was a well-groomed middle-aged woman. Her hair was neatly tied back into a bun. She was overly thin, with sunken cheeks. The black Mongolian winter gown intensified her grave facial expression.

"Your child has the fate of a nun. If she does marry, she will die." He rolled his cloudy eyes up and down as he went on.

I looked at my mother, and she looked at me. I wore two ponytails. My cheeks were hurting from the cold. I felt clumsy in the traditional Mongolian winter gown. Inner Mongolia was subject to long, cold winters with harsh blizzards. After a severe cold night, some homeless people were frozen to death in the street.

"This is the only child I have. What am I going to do? I have had poor health ever since I had the child, and won't be able to have another one. Good Heavens, what am I going to do?" my mother kept murmuring to herself.

"There could be a fix," the fortune-teller suggested. "Go to the temple and appeal to the master for help. Whenever people have problems, they always seek his protection."

"Thank you so much!" my mother said. "That's what I am going to do."

She reached into her winter gown with her skinny, sparrowlike hand, and pulled out a few coins. After counting carefully, she handed them to the fortune-teller and thanked him once more.

My mother grabbed my hand and wobbled on her tiny bound feet to find the old priest. For centuries, from the tender age of ten or earlier, it had been the practice that girls would have their feet wrapped tightly in bandages to prevent them from growing. Adult women therefore had extremely tiny feet, on which they could only walk with slow, tottering steps that were considered to be graceful. In modern days, people regard the practice as barbaric, a way for a male-dominated society to control women by physically disabling them. My mother often told me how painful it was to have had her feet bound when she was eleven. Deformed feet and intense pain and suffering came not only from the foot-binding process, but from its aftermath as well. Her four small toes were pressed downward toward the sole of her feet. The toenails would dig into the flesh causing excruciating pain or possible infection if they weren't trimmed properly. At the turn of the century, three things had become symbols of the nation's corruption: foot binding for women, wearing a queue for men, and opium consumption.

Several factors could have contributed to how I got away from having my own feet bound. When I approached the proper age, the custom was no longer in vogue; even though my parents belonged to the Han, China's main nationality, they were deeply influenced by "barbarians" like the Mongolians and the Manchus, who didn't have the foot-binding custom. Also my mother constantly suffered from health problems; she didn't have the energy to force me into things like that.

"No man is going to marry you if you have a pair of big feet," my mother often told me. In the old days, on the wedding day, when the new bride arrived in a sedan, her head would be covered by a red handkerchief and her feet would be the only thing the bridegroom could see. If he saw a pair of tiny bound feet, he would be very happy, even before he saw the face of the bride.

My mother didn't have a name. Since her family name was Yang, she was just addressed as Li Yang Shi — Mrs. Li Yang — her husband's surname plus her family name. She grew up in Chifeng. She was very outspoken, quite the opposite of my father Li Guorong, a man of few words. They were both born at the turn of the twentieth century, an extremely tumultuous period in history, as I've said — a time of foreign invasions, peasant uprisings, and warlords. This was when the Chinese empire was declining, half of its territory in the hands of foreign aggressors.

Before Europeans arrived in Asia, China, the Central Kingdom, considered itself to be the center of the universe, surrounded by inferior barbarians. While the dragon was sleeping during the eighteenth century, Europe had gone through an industrial revolution and before the Central Kingdom realized what was happening, enemies armed with modern weapons were already at the gate. After the First Opium War (1839–1842), China's rigid "closed door policy" ended and the country opened up to Western trade and Christian missionaries. The main trade was opium, introduced into China around the seventh century and originally used only as medicine. The Portuguese who occupied Macao taught the Chinese how to smoke it for recreation. Then the British introduced opium primarily grown in India to correct a trade deficit with China since there was little the Chinese needed from the West. Millions of Chinese became addicts of opium, which was known as "foreign mud."

Years later, the Taiping Rebellion (Heavenly Kingdom of Great Peace 1851–1864) broke out. It was one of the largest peasant uprisings in history led by Hong Xiuquan, who formulated an eclectic ideology combining the ideals of pre-Confucian utopianism with Protestant beliefs, aiming to overthrow the Qing Dynasty. Hong claimed to be the younger brother of Jesus Christ in order to gain legitimacy as the leader. Ironically, the rebellion was put down by Westerners, whom the rebels considered their brothers in Christ.

For the nation's survival, Emperor Guangxu, who was supported by a group of progressive scholar-reformers, issued a series of reforms aimed at sweeping social changes. The reform known as the Hundred Days' Reform only lasted 103 days — from June 11 to September 21, 1898 — before it was put down by the Empress Dowager Cixi, the strong-willed woman who dominated China for nearly half a century. Under her rule, the official incompetence and corruption of the Qing court reached its peak. To please the Empress, the devoted staff diverted funds intended for the navy to instead build a new Summer Palace to replace the old one which had been looted and burned down by the allied forces of British and French during the Second Opium War (1856–1860). My father was born in 1897, a year before the Hundred Days' Reform. He was originally from Luoyang, Henan Province. No one knew when his family moved to Chifeng or why.

In 1900, the year my mother was born, the anti-foreign and anti-Christian movement was started by the Society of Righteousness and Harmony. Westerners called them "Boxers" because they practiced martial arts and believed that they were invincible to bullets. Churches were burned, many missionaries and Chinese Christians were killed. The mystical Boxers were suppressed by allied troops of the eight foreign powers — Great Britain, France, Germany, Austria, Italy, Japan, Russia, and the United States.

Failure of reform from the top and the fiasco of the Boxers convinced many Chinese that the only solution was outright revolution, in order to get rid of the old system and establish a new one. The revolutionary leader Sun Yat-sen (1866–1925), who is considered to be the father of modern China by Nationalists and Communists alike, aimed to overthrow the Qing Dynasty, reunify a China beset with warlords, and establish a republic. On February 12, 1912, the last emperor, child Pu Yi, was abdicated. Afterward, there were a couple of unsuccessful attempts to restore the monarch. Among them were Yuan Shikai, who claimed himself as emperor in 1915, but whose imperial dream was short-lived; and Zhang Xun, who two years later in 1917, tried to reestablish the Qing Dynasty and failed. Old traditions die hard.

In July 1921, the Communist Party was formed by only twelve people including Mao. By the year I was born, 1926, the Communist Party had grown to sixty thousand members. The Nationalist Party, led by Sun Yat-sen, had forged an alliance with the fledging Communist Party during the early 1920s. After Sun died in 1925, the leadership of the Nationalist Party was transferred to Chiang Kai-shek, who never liked the Communists and in 1927 ordered the Nationalists to turn on their allies in a savage bloodbath that left thousands dead. This act resulted in the Chinese Civil War, which lasted until 1950.

In 1934, annihilation campaigns were waged against the Communists, forcing the Red Army to set on the epic Long March of some 12,500 kilometers. The Long Marchers didn't seem to have a specific direction, but with Chiang Kai-shek's army at their tail, they didn't stop for one year. They started from the south, headed southwest, and then north, until reaching Yan'an, Shaanxi Province, northwest China, where Mao lived in a cave for many years. Out of 100,000 soldiers in the beginning of the retreat, there were only 8,000 survivors. Among them was Deng Xiaoping, who became the paramount leader after Mao's era ended. However, over the next few years, the number of Communist Party members grew rapidly due to internal and external reasons, the most significant being the Japanese invasion. Mao Zedong made it through the

Nationalists' annihilation and the power struggles within the Communist Party during the Long March, and consolidated his position, gaining unchallenged command of the party.

While the Civil War went on, the Japanese were stepping up their control of Manchuria, the richest part of China in resources and industry. In 1932, the Japanese set up the last emperor Pu Yi, as puppet head of the new state of Manchukuo — Manchu country. In March 1933, Japanese invaded Chifeng and drove the Nationalists out of the city. Soon Manchu country expanded to eastern Inner Mongolia. As the Japanese military expanded in the region, Chiang Kai-shek's Nationalists insisted on the policy of "unity before resistance" and were more preoccupied with anti-Communist annihilation than with fighting the Japanese.

The *lao yie miao* temple the fortune-teller had mentioned was on the east side of the city. It was about a ten-minute walk from our home. *Lao ye miao*, is also called *guan di miao*. Guan Di is Guan Yu, a loyal and honorable general during the Three Kingdoms Period almost two thousand years ago. After he died, temples were erected to honor him. Over time he has been deified. The concept for an ordinary man to become a deity was common through Chinese history. Guan Yu is still widely worshipped today as an original Chinese deity, a Bodhisattva in Buddhism, and a guardian deity in Taoism. He is also highly regarded in Confucianism. He is also worshipped as the God of War and the God of Wealth. This is not contradictory in a Chinese religious system which blends various ancient philosophies and religions.

The temple only opened to worshippers on the first and fifteenth of every lunar month. On either side of the temple sat tall flagpoles, each placed in a solid stone base. I had to lift my head straight up to see the pointed top of the pole which was made of copper. The base of the pole was so wide that I couldn't even put my arms around it. It was the biggest temple in the city. A bright red, two-pieced gate opened inward. A large decorative copper ring on each side served as handles. The walls surrounding the temple were built with dark green bricks. After passing the gate, I saw an enormous incense burner in the middle of the spacious front yard. Inside the temple were all kinds of statues of people and horses. The crowds from the town and countryside came to "kowtow" and to burn incense or yellow-colored paper, called *biao*, as an offering. The whole yard was full of choking smoke.

On entering the temple, I came upon a frightening red-faced and long-toothed statue.

"Look, Mother, he can move his arms, even blink his eyes," I shouted. "The horse is moving too!" I was fascinated by all the looming mysterious figures.

While turning around, I was startled by a ferocious black-faced figure. I screamed in terror and ran out of the sacred place.

Later, when I had calmed down and returned, my mother spoke with the old priest. He listened to the tragic story, while stroking his long gray beard. "This is a very unfortunate situation," he said.

"I beg you, master, I heard that you have a solution to everything. There has to be something you can do so solve the problem, please." My mother put her palms together before her chest.

"There is a solution, but . . ." the kind-looking master said.

"Master, this is my only daughter, I'll do anything."

"Alright, I normally don't do this. But I'll make an exception this time for you. When is her birthday?"

"Lunar December 14."

"Buy a paper dummy in the market and dress it exactly like your daughter, and also buy a five-pound pig head, a three-pound chicken, and an eight-pound steamed bun. Come back here with your daughter on lunar December 14th."

✪

My mother devoutly believed in the master's solution. To raise the money for the items the priest needed, she had to pawn some of her earrings and ring, which had been her dowry at the time of her marriage. Three days before my birthday, we headed to the market.

I always got very excited in the market. The market square was in the city center, not far from where we lived. It was swarming with people. Vendors were crying their wares — everything from dried mushrooms to live chickens. It was close to the traditional New Year and people were already busy shopping. My mother couldn't walk as fast as I could and she often stopped to catch her breath. For a moment, I had the impression that she was going backward on her small bound feet. I was way ahead of her.

"Slow down, Qunying. I don't want to lose you in the crowd," she yelled. She was afraid to let me out of her sight. Rumor said that the Japanese captured people in order to use them in horrible experiments and they had some kind of nerve drug that could turn people into zombies who would do whatever they were told. I heard that many people had mysteriously gone missing, especially those from the countryside. I'd often heard my mother tell these terrifying stories. I just assumed that she was trying to scare me so I wouldn't go out to play by myself.

Accompanied by the deafening throb of gongs, a prisoner was dragged into the market for execution. As usual, the convict would first be paraded through the busy city streets before being executed. While the convict was escorted through the streets, many shopkeepers offered him liquor and food in front of their stores. The convict did not hesitate to enjoy one last moment of pleasure before death.

Japanese soldiers carried rifles, formed a circle in the center of the market square and pointed the shiny bayonets at the spectators. I was too small to see anything. Some children climbed onto trees to get a better look, but instead I climbed up onto a wagon that was parked by the street. The convict, who was tied up with a rope around his mouth, was kneeling down in the center of the circle. The executioner raised his sharp Japanese knife and swiftly chopped off the convict's head. Blood gushed and spurted high into the air as the head separated from the convict's neck and rolled away from the still-erect body. A buzz went through the mass of spectators who were watching with exhilaration.

In shock, I tumbled off the wagon and hit the ground very hard. For many nights I was unable to sleep well, because every time I closed my eyes, the scene of the rolling head and gushing blood would replay itself in my mind.

My mother bought a paper dummy from a shop. The shop made human figures, carriages and horses out of paper for customers to burn as offerings to the dead. Human figures were symbols of servants, and carriages or horses meant transportation. Those things were supposed to be used by the dead in the underworld.

She also bought a pig head and a chicken. The pig head weighed more than eight pounds, so she had to cut some of it off to achieve the exact five-pound weight that the priest had specified. She made an enormous-looking eight-pound steamed bun and dressed the paper dummy with my clothes to make it look as similar as possible to me. After preparing everything within three days, we set off for the temple on my birthday.

The ritual was performed in the yard at noontime. A long bench was placed in front of me. The paper dummy, the food offerings, the master, and I were all on one side of the bench. My mother was waiting nervously on the other side. The ritual began with the priest's incantations. Then he set the paper dummy on fire.

"Jump over the bench!" the priest said to me.

He gave me a rough slap on the back of my head that I still remembered many years later. After I crossed over to the other side of the bench, my mother grabbed my hand and dragged me out of the sacred place.

"Don't look back," the priest shouted. "The problem is solved. The child will live to be a hundred years."

While stepping out through the gate, I was still thinking about the food we had left behind.

Rat — the First Sign of the Horoscope

When I first started school at the age of seven, I was taught the *Three Character Classic* and *Hundred Family Surnames*, in the old traditional private school called *si su*. *Three Character Classic* was written in three character verses, short and simple so young children could memorize it and learn many common words and the fundamentals of Confucian morality. We were made to recite the whole text, even though we didn't necessarily understand the contents. We read loudly and moved our heads in rhythms. We had to recite in front of the teacher standing straight with both hands behind our backs. If we made a mistake, the teacher would punish us by smacking our palms with a ruler or making us stand for a long time. But it did make students pay more attention. I still remember clearly the first four verses: "People at birth, Are naturally good. While their natures are similar, Their habits make them different."

The Hundred Family Surnames — containing more than five hundred Chinese surnames — was also for the beginners. The first four surnames Zhao, Qian, Sun, and Li are believed to have been derived from the imperial families. In grade two, I learned the *Thousand Character Classic,* a poem used as a primer for teaching young children. *The Four Books and The Five Classics* outlined the ethics of society and government as well as codes for personal conduct, and were for more advanced students. When I got to grade three, we started to learn *Analects of*

Confucius — one of the *Four Books*, but it wasn't long before it was banned in school due to the Japanese occupation.

In 1937, the Japanese invaded China proper from their base in Manchuria and committed atrocities against innocent civilians. It was December when the Japanese entered the city of Nanjing and unleashed hideous violence and cruelty that were unparalleled in modern history. Unarmed civilians were tortured, raped, and killed. According to a median of various estimates, 260,000 civilians were massacred in this city alone. That was when the Communists and Nationalists hastily formed an alliance for the second time against the common enemy — Japan.

There were more than four hundred traditional private schools in the Chifeng area in 1930, but their numbers diminished after the Japanese occupation and many of them were converted into public schools that taught about Japanese culture and custom aimed to assimilate the Chinese people. Japanese became the official language while the Chinese language was forbidden in school.

Since a Japanese inspector only came to school to check up on the students once a week, many Chinese teachers, who resented the education aimed at enslavement, were reluctant to teach Japanese and secretly taught Chinese in the class when the inspector was away. When he came to school we would quickly hide our Chinese textbooks. I remember clearly the day when the inspector, a middle-aged, short, vicious-looking man with whiskers, came to check up on us. He rounded us up in the school playground, made us form a line, then pulled out one student at a time to recite the Japanese textbook. He made me walk in a straight line and followed right behind with a rattan stick in his hand. When I made a mistake, the inspector cracked his stick across my legs numerous times and the welts became swollen at once. Several boys were severely beaten that day. I returned home crying, but my mother insisted that I finish elementary school.

I had more interest in watching opera than in going to school. Because I had learned a few Japanese words, an old Japanese doorkeeper at the opera house often let us kids in without tickets. The most common show was Beijing opera. The front rows were always reserved for the rich and the Japanese. When the actors arrived in the city, their first night's performance was called "fire cannon." If they were successful, they could stay and perform for several years. But if they failed, people would fling watermelon rinds and nutshells onto the stage, and the actors would gather up all their belongings and flee the town that same night. In Beijing opera, the characters follow rigid stylized movements. There can't be one step more or one step less and even the motion of the figures has to be perfect, otherwise the experienced fans would notice the slight difference and create a disturbance. Famous actors were highly paid and didn't appear on stage every night. There was a very well-known actor with the nickname White Peony. He always played the female roles and dressed like a woman even when he was not on the stage.

I graduated from elementary school when I was twelve years old. Miss Zhu, my Chinese teacher, was very fond of me because I was a tomboy, very different from other girls in the school. She came to our home and talked to my parents. She wanted me to continue to learn Chinese secretly. I resumed study of *The Great Learning* and *The Analects of Confucius*. For the next three years, I read the texts at home and once a week I went to the school to recite in front of Miss Zhu. She also taught me *shufa* — a calligraphy that uses soft pointy ink brushes to write Chinese characters. This was considered a basic skill for the Chinese literati. To practice calligraphy I needed Four Treasures of the Study — ink brush, inkstick, ink-stone and paper. Before each elaborate session, I first prepared by adding some water into the inkstone in which I ground the inkstick (made of solidified ink) until the mixture became dark and thick. Then I placed a transparent paper over Miss Zhu's writings, and was ready to practice by tracing them. I dipped my brush in the inkstone, smoothed it out several times to get rid of excessive ink, and then carefully traced each stroke of the characters. When I showed my writing to Miss Zhu, she would make a check mark on the characters I wrote well, and circle the ones I needed more practice on. Later, my additional education would change the course my life would take.

The Chinese New Year of 1943 was fateful for me. I was about seventeen. "I want to go out to play," I said to my mother who was busy cooking.

"I told you many times you can't go out by yourself — it's dangerous," my mother said.

"But it's New Year's Eve; all the kids are playing outside."

"Quit bothering me. Don't you see I'm busy? Kids are not allowed to talk too much at New Year — it's bad luck."

"Why do you cook so much in one night, Mother?" I asked.

"Why do you ask so many questions? It's the custom. People are not supposed to cook anything on New Year's Day. Cooking raw food on New Year's Day is very bad luck and things can go wrong for the whole year. And no more questions! Kids may slip up and say something stupid and cause bad luck for the whole year."

My mother always avoided using words like "dead," "ghost," or "kill" during the New Year celebration, because she considered these words to be very ominous. She refrained from saying "dead fish" or "dead chicken" and instead replaced the word "dead" with "still."

"I think we should spend more money on new clothes, not so much on food," my mother said to my father. "We are wearing old clothes for the New Year. People will laugh at us."

"What's the use if we wear new clothes and go hungry?" my father said.

"At least we'll look decent."

"Every year at this time we have an argument over this."

"I can make some extra money making cloth shoes for the neighbors," my mother said. Since she had a pair of small bound feet, my mother had to make cloth shoes for herself. She produced them for others too, and was also very skilled at creating winter shoes for men, selling them for as much as two or three yuan a pair. Neighbors often came to buy shoes from her. It usually took her about three to four days to complete one pair. Like many women in the past, from a young age she had learned this traditional handicraft that had been around for thousands of years. Purchasing shoes in stores wasn't an option either because of the availability or the high price. I often watched my mother during her elaborate shoemaking sessions. First she would make the soles of the shoes by firmly stitching with thread many small pieces of leftover cloth from clothes making. This was the most difficult and time-consuming process. They also called the cloth shoes "thousand layer sole," because there were so many layers of cloth being used. It was very hard to sew through the layers of cloth by hand, so she had to drill a hole with an awl before she could put the thread through with a needle. She usually made one sole with hundreds of stitches. Then she would sew the uppers — usually a black color — and the soles together to complete the work. The cloth shoes were very soft, comfortable, and breathable. It was considered very elegant when a woman wore the white-soled black upper cloth shoes with a traditional *qipao* gown.

The room was saturated with cooking smoke and the smell of oily food. During the New Year, delicacies including chicken and fat pork, soaked in an oily broth, were served along with rarities like vegetables. I became so overwhelmed by the amount of food, which I wouldn't see normally, that I lost my appetite.

Our one-bedroom, one-living-room apartment was simply decorated with some old furniture. The most important pieces were two long dressers with drawers and had a mirror hanging above them. A cast-iron stove, fueled by a big chunk of coal sold by vendors from a nearby coal mine, provided not only heat in the severely cold winter but also the cooking fire.

As they did every New Year, residents placed a layer of wheat straw over the yard of the shared compound. When stepped on, the straw would make a crunching sound, as if, perhaps, to welcome the coming year. Families also placed an oil lamp on either side of their doors.

We rented our apartment from a rich midget landlord who was nicknamed Big Head Zhu because he possessed an extremely large head compared to his small body. He owned the entire huge residential compound. There were about thirty houses around a rectangular-shaped courtyard, and it took me a long time just to walk around it. The roofs of the old houses were tiled in dark green and each corner was decorated with dragons. The residents were mostly workers or small street vendors like my father. Everyone kept to themselves. I don't remember any neighbor ever visiting us. In fact, the residents didn't even talk to each other.

Landlord Zhu had four wives. He had almost lost his huge head recently. The Japanese wanted to buy his head because they said there was a key inside it that could open the Red Mountain, which was supposedly filled with treasure. I was always fascinated by the Red Mountain in the northeast corner of our ancient city and admired the flaming color reflected from its red granite. Luckily, Big Head Zhu had money and power on his side so, in the end, even the Japanese couldn't succeed in acquiring this large prize.

After the New Year's Eve supper, I rested my head on my mother's leg as she gently stroked my hair. I could hear the sound of firecrackers and the shouting of the children outside. I felt that even though I didn't have new clothes for the New Year, I was still the happiest child in the world.

Everything would have been all right if I hadn't talked too much that New Year's Eve. Many years later, I still wondered what had gotten into me. That one silly question, which I always regretted saying, changed my entire life.

"Why haven't I ever dressed in white clothes like others do?" I suddenly asked my mother out of the blue.

Little did I know that white clothes were a symbol of mourning. After seeing my mother's face turn pale, I sensed that I had made a huge mistake.

"Go to sleep," she said, patting me on the head. "Kids are not allowed to speak too much at New Year."

Then, for the remainder of the night, she kept chanting, "Kids say innocent things. Gods forgive her. Kids say innocent things . . ."

Tormented by what I had said, my mother didn't sleep well that night. The next morning, I was excited and got up early. It was New Year's Day!

A huge rat emerged from my mother's quilt on that New Year's morning. Armed with brooms, my father and I embarked on a rat-hunting adventure. The rat dashed out of the bedroom and into the living room where I hit at it with the broom several times and missed it. It hid under the cupboard so I used the handle of the broom to scare it out. When it finally came out from under the cupboard, I took careful aim and hit it with all my strength. There was a blood-curdling shriek — but not from the rat. It came from the bedroom. I ran in and found my mother sitting straight up in bed, her eyes staring ahead in horror.

After we killed the rat, my mother started acting strangely. She swore that it was all to do with the fact that she was born in the year of rat, according to Chinese astrology. The traditional lunar calendar was based on a twelve-year cycle, and each year was named after a certain animal. One version of the legend has it that Buddha invited all the animals to come to him before he departed from the Earth. Only twelve came to bid him farewell. As a reward he named each of the twelve years after each animal in the order they had arrived. First came the rat. Yet another legend has it that the Jade Emperor, heaven's ruler, asked to see the Earth's twelve most interesting animals, was impressed by the rat's cleverness, and awarded it first place. Chinese take the symbolic animals very seriously, and especially did in the old days. Even marriages were arranged around it so there wouldn't be conflicts between the bride and bridegroom. People believed that the animal ruling the year in which a person was born determined his or her personality and fortune.

"I'm a rat, and now I have revealed my true self. My days are numbered," my mother said sadly, as if her soul had already left her body.

My mother's illness had gotten progressively worse over time. In the early fall of that same year, she was critically ill and became bedridden. I was afraid to look at her because she used to be skinny and now she had suddenly become swollen all over, barely opening her eyes. We didn't have the money to get her in to see a doctor at the hospital. There was a big hospital in the city, called Jing Long Hospital. It was privately owned, very expensive, and staffed with some Japanese doctors.

A few days before my mother passed away, I heard a bell ring in the street. A "wild doctor" — a medicine man who wandered through the streets — was ringing it to attract customers. The medicine men were also called *guo lu xian sheng* — passing-by doctors. My father ran out to find the doctor and brought him home. The doctor had a long gray beard and wore a traditional robe. On his shoulder, he carried a *dalian* — a long, rectangular bag sewn up at both ends, full of all kinds of herbs.

Everyone in the room seemed to stop breathing when the doctor was taking my mother's pulse. I looked at the doctor and tried to guess what his diagnosis might be. His face was blank. After the examination, he sighed. We didn't dare to ask any questions for fear that, if we did, something would go terribly wrong. He brought out some herbal medicine and gave my father strict instructions to follow. Over the months, many wild doctors came into our home, and a lot of money went out for medicines that had no effect. But every time a new doctor arrived, we would get our hopes up.

My father was busy boiling the herbs he received from the wild doctor. Soon the room was filled with the strong smell of medicine — the familiar aroma I had been used to for many months now since my mother had become ill. He followed the medicine man's instructions very carefully. He placed the herbs and several cups of water in an earthenware cooking vessel, covered it very tightly, and boiled the mixture over a low flame for five hours until half of the liquid evaporated. After that, he would strain it through cheesecloth and divide the decoction into two portions. My mother would take one in the morning and one in the evening on an empty stomach. The full treatment was six months. One course was ten days. And there were usually ten days between each course.

"My daughter, I'm dying," she whispered in a very weak voice. "What are you going to do after I die?"

"Why do people have to die? Where do you go when you die?" I was crying.

"My child, Yanwang, the ruler of the underworld, has an enormous book of names and lists all the people who live on Earth. Every day, Yanwang selects a number of names from his book; he instructs his servants, who are armed with ropes, to capture these people, and return them to hell." My mother gazed at me with swollen eyes that could hardly stay open.

Two days before she died, we made dumplings for her to eat. According to the old custom, the number of the dumplings she could eat represented the number of days she had left. She ate one and a half. My mother died the day after, on an afternoon in lunar September 1943. She was only forty-three years old.

I had to perform the ritual of smashing a clay basin into pieces against the ground to officially begin the funeral. Then the lengthy march to the burial site started. A horse-drawn carriage carried the coffin, while I walked in front with a long narrow funeral streamer made of paper in my hand. It was believed that when people died, the spirit would leave the body and rise up into space. The purpose of the funeral streamer was to call back the spirit of the dead. Because I was short, the streamer dragged on the ground around my feet as I paraded down the street dressed in white mourning clothes.

All the relatives attended the funeral. I didn't cry. In fact, I felt as though I was in a daze. I had to be led by a cousin. I couldn't even remember how I had walked eight miles to the destination.

We couldn't afford to buy a burial plot for my mother. The only alternative was Nanyuanzi, eight miles south from the town, a place where most people left their loved ones' coffins above the ground. Instead of burying the coffins deep in the earth, they lay them on the surface, sealing them with a thin coat of mud, which was a less costly procedure than full burial. Afterward, I stood the funeral streamer in front of my mother's grave.

If no one attended the "grave" for a certain period of time, the coffin would most likely be removed by caretakers. If not, it would decompose within two or three years anyway. In 1999, more than fifty years after, I placed a call to a wool sweater factory in Chifeng by chance and asked about the burial spot. I was told that everything had changed. High-rises had been built over it.

I didn't understand why my mother had to suffer such an ill fate. Shortly after my mother passed away, I went to consult the same blind fortune-teller that she and I had once visited. After some rolling and blinking of his muddy eyes, he said that my mother had either passed away or, if she was alive, she was seriously ill. I was very surprised.

"How could you possibly know that?" I asked.

"You *ke* your mother," he said.

"What does *ke* mean?"

"*Ke* means to oppose or conflict with. It all originated from the I Ching, the ancient divination."

"Do you mean people may be in conflict even though they are close to each other?"

"That's usually the case."

✪

On the Ghost Festival, almost a year after my mother had passed away, I followed the procession of people to the river that flowed beside the Red Mountain. Every year, on the night of lunar July 15, people would gather at the riverbank to display lanterns of all sorts to commemorate their dead relatives. Even the ladies from rich families, who rarely ventured out of their homes, arrived in horse-drawn carriages with awnings on them. The Japanese women, wearing kimonos, also made an appearance at the ceremony. I placed a lantern in the river and said a prayer. It slowly floated down the river and joined the rest, which together resembled a dragon.

I didn't return home until two o'clock in the morning. The Japanese women, impressed by the few Japanese words that I had learned in school, took a liking to me and gave me a ride home in their vehicle. When I got back, my aunt was waiting for me unexpectedly.

"I have never seen a girl go wild like a boy," my aunt said. "I was really worried about you. It's dangerous out there."

"There are many people outside," I said. "Where's my father?" I could tell something was wrong because my aunt looked very nervous.

"You have to live with us for a while. The Japanese are rounding people up as slaves. I heard that people rarely survive. Your father has to go hide," she said to me.

"How long is it going to be?"

"I don't know."

"Where did he go?"

"I have no idea. But as soon as it's safe, he'll come back to get you."

My father fled in a hurry and didn't even have time to say goodbye. He only took a quilt with him. I never saw him again. Years later, I made several guesses about what had happened to him. One thought was that he had been caught by the Japanese and hadn't survived the grueling life of an enslaved laborer. The second guess was that he had joined the Communist Eighth Route Army and possibly had died on the battlefield. I didn't think that there was any possible chance that my father would have become a bandit, since he had always been an honest and timid person. I have since read the historical record of Chifeng, and found out that in one incident the Japanese rounded up over a hundred slave laborers and forced them to construct military fortifications and a road near Chifeng area. After the projects were complete, the laborers were mysteriously disappeared. The truth was only revealed in 1969 by a former slave laborer, a sole survivor: over one hundred laborers were killed by the Japanese. Soon afterward, two mass graves were found. One contained over forty human skulls; the other held many skeletons one on top of the other. That was the possible fate my father might have suffered and the worst case scenario I could have imagined. I have never had closure on this matter.

So I took all our belongings, which consisted of mostly furniture and some savings my father had left me, and went to live with my aunt. My aunt had a fairly big family: her husband, two daughters, and a mother-in-law and father-in-law who reluctantly took me in. They saw me as a burden, especially due to the fact that I was a girl. I was already about eighteen and there were not many prospects for me. Men and women were not equal by any means and in those days it was very difficult for a woman to find a job, even if she had a higher education. Girls were not encouraged to study. Like Confucius said: "Ignorance is a virtue of women." So not many girls had any ambition. My aunt was just a housewife. My cousin, who was a couple of years older than me, dropped out of junior high school, had no job, and was doing embroidery at home. She had a mild temperament and was at the age of marriage. From her I learned to do needlework, but I was never good at it. All I could do to earn my keep was to help my aunt with the housework. In my spare time, I would read books — mostly Japanese propaganda materials, or play with my younger cousin and watch operas. I was hoping that someday the opportunity would present itself when I wouldn't have to depend on others.

3

The Eighth Route Army

On a summer afternoon in 1945, I heard a loud noise in the street. I wanted to go out to take a look.

"Don't go out, it's dangerous out there. I just heard that the *lao mao zi* are coming," my aunt said to me. I had been living with my aunt for a couple of years by then.

"Who are the *lao mao zi?*" I asked.

"Russians! People are saying that they raped women and did other bad things. Some young women painted their faces black with ashes from underneath the cooking pots, dressed in ragged clothes and stayed home all day to avoid trouble." *Lao mao zi* was a derogatory local slang name for the Russians who had invaded the northeast region many times in the past.

"I haven't been out for many days, I just want to take quick look at what's going on," I said.

"Just be careful, don't be long. I heard that in wintertime, the *lao mao zi* dig a hole in the ice and jump right in to have a bath. They are animals," my aunt said.

That was the first time I saw a tank. The Russian soldiers stood on the tanks with guns in their hands. The Soviet Red Army had stormed in from the north border to fight the Japanese. The Soviet Union decided to enter the Second World War's Pacific Theater within three months after the end of the war in Europe. On August 8, 1945, Soviet Union mobilized 1.5 million soldiers, launched the massive Operation August Storm (or the Battle of Manchuria) against the Japanese, and won a decisive victory. Transbaikal Front — one of the three Red Army fronts that invaded western Manchkuo — liberated Chifeng. The Soviets' Operation August Storm, together with the two atomic bombs dropped on Japan, forced the Japanese to surrender. Korea, a former Japanese colony, was divided into two parts along the 38th parallel after the Soviet Army invaded northern Korea while the Americans occupied the south. This invasion became a precursor to the Korean War five years later.

The Soviet Army maintained very strict discipline. The soldiers who had committed the rapes my aunt spoke of were all lined up and shot. In total, twelve were shot in Chifeng alone. Locals considered the Russians to be worse than the Japanese. Among the liberators, was also the shabbily clothed Chinese Communist Eighth Route Army.

People were cheering in the crowded street, "The Japanese have surrendered!"

I spotted dead bodies. They were everywhere in the streets. Many Japanese soldiers and civilians had committed suicide with knives or taken overdoses of opium. Numerous Japanese women and children were also abandoned during the chaos. The old Japanese doorkeeper at the opera house held an opium brick in his hand and told people in his broken Chinese: "I finished. I take this."

The citizens ran in all directions, wild with joy. A lot of people rushed to the opium-trading warehouse to loot the opium bricks without realizing that the warehouse was surrounded by high voltage power lines. Many got electrocuted, and some who lacked any knowledge of electricity tried to rescue the dying men, but they ended up getting electrocuted themselves one after another. The Japanese had encouraged people to grow opium and had collected it as taxes in order to finance the war and poison the body and mind of the Chinese.

I followed the frenzied crowds to the lao ye miao temple. Less than a month earlier, one of the two flagpoles on the side of the temple had fallen without warning, knocked down houses nearby, and killed several people. At the base of the fallen pole was a two-meter deep hole that was filled with snakes. Citizens considered the fall of the flagpole to be an omen that Japanese rule would soon be coming to an end. On August 6 and 9, 1945, Americans dropped two atom bombs in Japan, one on Hiroshima and the other on Nagasaki. Shortly afterward, Japan surrendered. When the war ended, an estimated 20 million Chinese had been killed by the Japanese.

Now, a month later, the Eighth Route Army was removing basket after basket of snakes from the hole, some of them dead and some still alive. They re-erected the flagpole in front of the temple, pouring concrete into the bases. At first the citizens were doubtful if the Communists had the mandate of heaven to accomplish such a task. Legend had it that these two poles were erected by a "Number One Scholar" — the title for the one who came first in the highest imperial examination — an ancient system in choosing government officials. The people in Chifeng believed that only the person with this achievement had the mandate of heaven to be able to set up the two huge flagpoles. After the pole was set up, the citizens became convinced that the Communists were there to stay. The Eighth Route Army not only set up the pole but also somewhat proved its legitimacy.

In the troop, I spotted a familiar face. It was my Chinese teacher, Miss Zhu. Previously she had once been arrested by the Japanese and tortured, but didn't admit she was an underground Communist. Now everyone knew that she really was a Communist. She became the mayor of Chifeng. She talked to me about women's liberation. "Women shouldn't depend on others and should be on their own," she said to me. I was greatly influenced by her.

"I saw Teacher Zhu in the street today," I said to my aunt. I'd had an exciting day and come home in the late evening. "She's a Communist."

"Where did you go for the whole day? I was worried about you," my aunt said.

"I want to join the Eighth Route Army, Auntie," I said. "Teacher Zhu has told me everything about it."

"They don't look like an army, more like a bunch of bandits," she said.

"They are helping the poor people," I told her.

The next day, Teacher Zhu came to our home and explained to my aunt about the Communist army. My aunt was happy for me to finally have an opportunity to become independent — she knew this was exactly what I wanted. Teacher Zhu told everybody that if they missed me they could just go to the army base a few miles away to visit me, and I could come back to see them. In reality, the army had a very strict discipline — it wasn't so easy to obtain a leave to visit a relative. I said goodbye to my aunt and joined the army at the age of nineteen. I was still wearing a traditional summer gown. I also brought with me a winter gown. My aunt gave me a pair of silver chopsticks with a chain link and told me that they would turn black when coming in contact with poison during a meal. I also brought my family photo album and a silver bracelet that my mother had left for me, but which I would never have a chance to wear in the army. When I arrived, they registered my age, address, family members, and property status. Then it was arranged that I would stay in a dormitory with several other female soldiers. On the third day, I was allotted an army uniform and said goodbye to civilian clothes. The first uniform I received was a muddy-colored mix of yellow and green. It had been dyed with diluted gunpowder. After a few washes, the uniforms would turn pale again and look even more terrible than ever. Since I had received some schooling, which basically meant I could write a few words and count some numbers, I was considered well educated among the soldiers and officers, who were mostly illiterates, unable to even recognize their own names in print. As a result, I became a bookkeeper in an ammunition factory of the 13th Brigade, and everyone treated me with great respect.

On lunar September 14, 1946, the moon shone brightly with a temperature of thirty below. Winter came earlier to Inner Mongolia than to many other places. I was at a meeting that evening. The literary teacher was talking about Marx and Lenin. He said the rich were getting richer, and the poor were getting poorer all because of the exploitation by the rich. With Communism everyone would have their share. No one would go hungry again. He explained that the Communists would overthrow the capitalists and landlords, confiscate their factories, businesses, lands, and properties, and then disperse them among workers and peasants. He talked about revolution. That was the first time I heard the word revolution — "geming" — transform or eliminate lives. It took me many years to understand its real meaning.

Suddenly, I heard gunshots. Without warning, the Nationalists raided the ammunition factory. After the Japanese had surrendered, the Civil War had resumed in earnest between the Nationalists and the Communists. The alliance between the Communists and Nationalists was flawed from the very beginning. Both parties regarded each other with suspicion.

We fled in such a hurry that my knapsack and some irreplaceable family photos of my parents and myself were all left behind. Many years later, I was to remember the long-lost childhood photo of myself at just two years old, wearing long ponytails. On the back of the photo was written: "Born in *zishi*, on lunar December 14, 1925, in Chifeng." *Zishi*, a period of time from 11 p.m. to 1 a.m., was part of the old method of tracking time. Since there was no clock in the house, they could only guess the time of my birth. Even now, I still insist upon celebrating my birthday on lunar December 14 according to the old calendar. Every year, my children have trouble figuring out my birth date, because each time it falls on a different day of January, and occasionally even in February.

After running a few miles, we caught up with a truck that was loaded with ammunition. Everyone was rushing into it. As I put my left leg up into the truck, I felt a sting in my right calf. It became numb for a moment but didn't hurt. After we came out of the city, I noticed that my right felt boot seemed sticky inside. "You got shot," someone said to me.

I reached down to my calf and felt something wet. It was blood, dark under the moonlight. The bullet had gone through my thick felt boot. I held my injured leg and started crying. "Don't cry. You'll be okay," a nurse said. She dressed the wound to stop the bleeding. Two weeks later when we got to Qiqihar, Heilongjiang Province in the Northeast, I was sent to a hospital where I had the bullet removed. Luckily, it didn't cause serious damage.

From October 1946 to mid 1947, we stayed in the Northeast to fight the bandits who ran rampant throughout the area. They robbed people and even in broad daylight kidnapped them for ransom. They would cut off a hostage's finger or ear, and send it to the family through a middleman to urge them to pay ransom more quickly. Many once-lawful people resorted to banditry. The reasons were very complicated, but the main reason was poverty, beginning during the worldwide Great Depression in the early thirties. The Civil War and Japanese invasion had compounded the problem, and banditry became epidemic throughout the country, especially in the northeast region where banditry had a long history. According to some estimates, in 1946 the number of bandits in the Northeast alone was between 90,000 and 130,000.

When the Japanese controlled the three provinces in the Northeast in the early thirties, the bandit situation became more complex. Many bands of bandits were anti-Japanese, while some were anti-Communist. Those who had a close relationship with the Nationalists were both anti-Japanese and anti-Communist. There were some brought over and incorporated into the Japanese forces. Adding to the confusion, the bandits were not steadfast in their stand. They would support the Japanese one day and side with the Communists the next. After the Japanese surrendered, Chiang Kai-shek incorporated some armed bandits into the Nationalist troops. In order for us to establish a base in the Northeast to fight the Nationalists, the first thing we had to do was to wipe out the banditry.

There were two particular bandit leaders we were chasing, one called Sister Liu and the other, Black Dragon. In the early spring, we reached "Snake Valley" at about eleven o'clock at night after a long march through rough mountain trails. My flesh crawled at the mere mention of the snakes. Everyone was exhausted, hungry, and thirsty, but despite a thorough search of the village, we could find absolutely no water. The villagers' water vat turned out to be empty. The well was also bone-dry and a ten-meter rope couldn't even reach the bottom. Every morning at four o'clock, the villagers would travel a long distance on ox carts to transfer water with wicker baskets sealed with mud. The strange thing was that the soil in this vicinity was very damp and spongy when stepped on, as if it contained water.

We settled into an enormous house that belonged to a landlord who had run away when he heard the Communists were coming. A dog still tied to a tree was barking at us. Inside, in the kitchen, we discovered a large pot brimming with cooked millet. When we lifted the cover off the pot, the delicious aroma filled the room, so we could tell that the landlord had escaped not long ago. No one touched the millet, because the army did not allow troops to take civilians' property. We attempted to eat our parched flour without a drop of water to wash it down. Some of us choked. Parched flour was the main food for us because it was light to carry and could be preserved for long periods of time without spoiling.

Some soldiers slept on the floor, while a few nurses and I slept on the *kong* bed, which was constructed of mud tiles and connected to the kitchen stove. The bed was warm and cozy but I was deadly afraid of snakes, so I tied my pants legs and cuffs with shoelaces and, as an added precaution, placed a towel over my mouth to prevent the slimy pests from crawling in. Even though I was exhausted, I still remained very alert. The snakes were slithering all over the bed and gave me goosebumps.

Next morning, the troop commenced efforts as it always did on arriving in a new place: tramped from house to house promoting the party's land reform rule and the policy of getting rid of bandits. Mao was aware of the important role of the peasants in establishing a base in the Northeast. Because the Soviet Revolution succeeded in the urban areas, Stalin had long dismissed Mao's rural guerrilla strategy. However, Mao was convinced that the Chinese urban workers were unable to lead the revolution because they made up only a small portion of China's population. Therefore, the revolution could only depend on the peasants, who were eighty percent of the population. His strategy was to establish bases in the rural areas and "encircle the cities from the countryside and then capture them." Land was the most important issue for the peasants who were ruthlessly exploited by landlords. Many peasant uprisings throughout history were land-related.

Mao had attempted a series of land reforms since the late twenties but for various reasons these reforms weren't thorough enough. To mobilize and win the support of the peasants in the Civil War, he launched an extensive land reform in May 1946, which confiscated landlords' acreage and redistributed it to peasants who tilled it. Supported by Communist armies, the oppressed peasants let out their indignation during violent mass rallies against the landlords. This strategy worked. This land reform was an important factor in how the Communists could first win the war in the countryside, then swiftly defeat the Nationalists in three short years.

At first, the villagers were afraid and avoided us. Whenever they caught a glimpse of the soldiers, they would scurry away quickly. At the time, the peasants in Snake Valley didn't grow food crops, but instead produced opium. All the villagers smoked opium, including the unmarried young women, whose parents had great difficulty finding them husbands because of their addiction. The young women never washed their faces, and whenever sweat ran down their cheeks, it would leave behind white streaks. To earn the villagers' trust, we helped the peasants plant opium in the spring. By July, the plants developed beautiful lotuslike flowers, and, in August, gourds grew after the flowers fell. When harvest season came, I was taught to cut the gourds with a knife. A milky white liquid flew out and soon turned black after being dried in the sun. The opium was then processed into bricks, which were said to be even more valuable than bars of gold.

Our work paid off. Slowly they began to trust us and provided us with plenty of crucial information. Some of the villagers searched the forests for family members who had joined the bandits, and persuaded them to turn themselves in. Many bandits showed up, handed in their weapons and confessed their crimes.

The runaway landlord was eventually apprehended. All his property, including land and houses, was divided among the villagers. The landlord was said to be a "despotic landlord" and possessed his own armed forces, called "village soldiers," who not only protected his own properties but also that of the whole village from bandit attacks. During the Anti-Japanese War, he had supported the Communists' fight against the Japanese by donating money, grain, and weapons. The villagers held a mass rally against the landlord, then dragged him around the village with a horse until the back of his skull fell off. He had several wives. His youngest wife was beaten to death. She was the prettiest, but, for some reason, the villagers hated her. His oldest wife was older than the landlord himself. She was a child bride and she had been married to him when he himself was just a few years old. Because the villagers didn't have "popular indignation" toward her, they gave her a house to live in and some other properties.

The landlord had been addicted to opium. After he died, a huge snake hung down from the roof of his house, half-dead. We figured that the snake might have been living on the roof for many years, becoming addicted to opium as the landlord smoked. Now with the landlord gone, the snake was experiencing withdrawal.

We finally captured the bandits, all twelve of them. After several days and nights we had chased down Sister Liu, who was waving a gun in each hand. By the time we finally caught up with her, she had lost a lot of blood from a gunshot wound in her leg. Soldiers dug twelve body-sized holes in the ground where the bandits were all lined up. They asked Sister Liu if she had any last words before they shot her.

"I lived a good life. I had the best clothes, and the best horses. I have no regrets. I'll reincarnate, and do it all over again," she said calmly.

All the twelve bandits were shot and fell right into the pits. After the execution, the soldiers began to march away, leaving the peasants to stay behind and bury the bodies. One bandit suddenly arose from his grave, blood and dust all over his face.

"Officers, spare me, please! I'm a good man. Spare me . . ." he yelled.

One soldier went back and shot him again, this time killing him. By mid 1947, the bandits were mostly wiped out. After the bandits were all taken care of, the villagers were overcome with gratitude. As the troop left the village, the villagers came out of their houses, kneeled down on the side of the streets and kowtowed to us.

"Thank you very much, you are heaven-sent. We'll never suffer at the hands of the bandits ever again," they said.

4

THE DOCTOR

WHILE I WAS AWAY with the troop, Chifeng changed hands many times. Often the Nationalists occupied the city during the day, the Communists took it over at night, and the Nationalists retook it the next day. In the summer of 1947, the Communists finally seized Chifeng.

A few months later, I returned to my hometown. The first thing I wanted was to find out if my father had returned. It was hard for me obtain a two-hour leave to go out of the military base alone; the Nationalist troops were just a couple hundred miles away from us and they could launch a counterattack at any time. I went to our old house to look for my father, but couldn't find him. No one had seen him. Some of the houses in the residential compound had been badly damaged during the war, and the landlord Big Head Zhu had disappeared. I was deeply saddened to see the house still standing but someone else living in it instead of my own family. I went back to my aunt's place a few blocks away. My father had never contacted her. My cousin had gotten married and my aunt wanted me to stay for supper, but I told her that I had to hurry back to the base. That was the only time I had visited her after I joined the army. It was also the last.

The Communist army took over the private Jing Long Hospital. It was the biggest hospital in the city. Some of the hospital staff ran away with the Nationalists. Others decided to stay. There were even some Japanese doctors who refused to go back to their own country and remained after the Japanese surrendered.

My office was just beside the Jing Long Hospital, and every day I could see doctors and nurses coming in and out of the hospital in their clean white overalls.

That was what I would like to do: be a doctor, not a bookkeeper. I didn't think I was the type who could sit in an office crunching numbers all day. That was not revolution. Revolution should be like a rainstorm, a blizzard, a hurricane, or blood and fire. To be a doctor is a sacred career. My mother would have been proud of me. I immediately applied for work in the hospital.

"I want to be a doctor," I said to Teacher Zhu.

"You never studied medicine. What can you do?" she asked.

"Well, I'm willing to learn to be a doctor," I said enthusiastically. "Now it has become the people's hospital and the poor can also have access to doctors. In the past, my mother couldn't afford to see a doctor in this hospital. If that had been now, she wouldn't have died."

"All right," Teacher Zhu said, after giving the matter some thought. "Why not start as a receptionist in the hospital and work your way up while you are learning?"

That was how I got started on my path to becoming a doctor. I had never stopped wondering what the real cause of my mother's death was. I suspected it was kidney disease. It made sense since her whole body had been swollen. Later, I would change my diagnosis to stomach disease.

At the beginning, just as Miss Zhu had suggested, I worked as a receptionist in the hospital, but, just a few short days later, I started learning how to give shots. It was said that because the Japanese had established some bacteriological warfare bases in northeast China, many epidemic diseases, especially the plague, became prevalent. At the time of their surrender, before escaping, the Japanese set free thousands of infected rats, causing widespread plague in the Northeast, which took hundreds of thousands of lives.

When I was young, I had heard that during the Japanese occupation, whenever the plague was detected, the Japanese soldiers would seal the infected village and douse the place with gasoline, burning it to the ground together with the dead and the living. Escape was impossible. Often they would burn down the nearby villages as well. After that, not a trace of any living thing could be spotted in a circumference of a hundred miles.

Soon I was not just a secretary. I followed the medical team everywhere. We sanitized the streets and houses, isolated the patients, encouraged people to kill rats, and administered vaccine shots in Chifeng and its suburbs. At first, the suspicious villagers were afraid to accept vaccine shots and hid their children away when the medical team arrived, either because they lacked trust in modern medicine or due to long-standing rumors that the Japanese were conducting experiments on humans. The Nationalists' propaganda also added to their distrust of the Communists. It took hard work to convince the villagers that we were there to help and that the vaccine was in their best interests. I acquired a new skill after being shown how to give a needle by a defected Japanese nurse. I was a little clumsy on the first day but the second day was better. The vaccine bottle was huge: one bottle was enough for two hundred people. Often I would give up to five hundred injections per day in a single village. The needles would be boiled and reused.

To dispose of those who had died from plague, we drenched the mountain of dead bodies with industrial alcohol and gasoline, then set them ablaze in an open field. For many years, the gruesome image of the dead, their arms and legs twisting in a sea of flames, along with the sizzling of burning flesh and foul stench, haunted me in my nightmares.

After the vaccination work was over, I learned to deliver babies, again from a Japanese doctor who had defected after the Japanese surrendered. The old, overweight doctor, who walked with a limp, could speak fluent Chinese and always politely addressed me as "Li san." He told me that at first he hadn't wanted to come to China, but he had been told by the Japanese government that it was his duty to do so. Now he didn't want to go back.

When the New Year arrived, I couldn't obtain a leave to celebrate with my aunt's family, so I worked during the holiday. The Japanese doctor and the nurses had nowhere to go either, so we got together to cook and make some dumplings. Just as we were going to sit down to have our New Year's Eve dinner, a woman came in, about to have her baby. After delivering the baby, we sat down at the table to try to finish our meal. I could hardly eat so soon after the dramatic scene of a childbirth. Then, once again, before we could even get started on our meal, another woman rushed in. In total, there were five women who had babies that night. The dishes had to be warmed up many times and it took us the whole night to finish eating.

Soon I got tired of the job and asked for a transfer to the operating room. After three months of training in the operating room, at the beginning of 1948, I joined the medical team of the Second Regiment of the 13th Brigade, as we moved out of the city. I wanted to say goodbye to my aunt but couldn't get permission for leave from the leaders. The reason I was given was that she wasn't my immediate family. I scribbled a note in a great hurry but was never able to find out if it was delivered to her or not. I eventually lost all contact with my hometown and have never returned since that day. The troop moved south to fight the Nationalists, further and further away from Chifeng. I had hoped that I would someday return, but it never materialized. I never heard from my aunt because I wasn't allowed to write letters, nor was there a mail system during the chaotic war; our troop moved to a different location every day. After liberation in 1949, I sent letters to my aunt but never received any response. By that time Chifeng had undergone great changes and I guessed that they might have moved to a new address.

Otherwise, even though my aunt was illiterate, my cousin could have read the letters to her.

The army attacked and seized many smaller cities along the way. The troop always marched at night. One night, while on the move, we crossed paths with the Nationalist troops without recognizing each other due to the darkness. We only found out they were enemies after exchanging passwords. A fierce battle broke out and when it was over we had caught several Nationalist officials. We were stationed on a mountain near Chengde City, which was still occupied by the Nationalists. Lights were strictly forbidden at night and we were always prepared for an enemy attack at any time. We lived in tents, using only grass as bedding. There were twelve soldiers in my squad including four women. In the daytime, we did exercises and literacy study. Since I had attended school before, I was assigned as literacy tutor. An older female soldier taught me how to weave sweaters. Villagers often let their sheep roam out on the mountain, which gave us the opportunity to gather up the wool they shed, then twist it into knitting wool with our hands. When we ran out of millet to eat, we headed down into the village at night to collect food. The villagers had nothing left, since the Nationalist soldiers had robbed them of food during the day. We stayed on the mountain for weeks before we moved on.

The Battle of Zunhua was the most brutal. So many soldiers died storming the heavily fortified high wall of the old Zunhua city that ladders were constructed with all the dead bodies from both the Nationalists and the Communists. I entered the town after the battle was over. We were told not to touch any food or drink in the warehouse because these supplies might have been poisoned by the Nationalists.

Since we were always on the move, our medical supplies would be carried by two mules. Bandages and medicines were in short supply, so we had to boil the used bandages and gauze in order to reuse them. The bandages were just plain white cloths, which, when needed in an emergency, were sometimes not sanitized. Iodine, alcohol, and anesthetic were considered to be extremely precious, used only when absolutely necessary. During the major battles, we could see fifty or sixty wounded soldiers a day. The most common treatment was to wash the wound with salt water, then wrap it up with a bandage. Because of the lack of medicine, we could often only watch the patients die. We simply weren't able to do anything. The soldiers with light wounds would be treated and immediately returned to the frontline whereas the ones requiring longer recovery times would be transferred to base hospitals that were also constantly moving; conditions weren't much better there.

Along the way, a clinic was set up in a villager's home, which had two long dressers that could be used as temporary sickbeds for patients. It was only a temporarily clinic. A few days after our clinic was set up, an unconscious soldier was carried in on a stretcher. He had been badly injured in a battle. For the first time, I assisted a surgeon during the operation. We had no other alternative but to cut off both his arms and legs. I tried to ignore the chilling sound of bones being cut through with a small copper saw. When the patient regained consciousness, and found he had lost all his limbs and had only his torso remaining, he became hysterical, refusing to eat or accept treatment.

"Get the hell out of here," he yelled when I approached him.

When I attempted to feed him, he tried to bite me. He missed, lost his balance, and couldn't turn over by himself. He struggled and swore with the most obscene words he could come up with in his Shanxi dialect.

A month later, the patient was sent back to his hometown. An official accompanied him home.

"What happened to him?" I asked the official when he came back a week later.

"His mother refused to accept her own son. She said that it wasn't her son because he hadn't looked like that when he had left home. 'What have you done to my son?' she said. I didn't know how to calm her down. I told her that revolution came with a cost. On the other hand, his wife vowed to take care of him for the rest of his life."

"What is he going to do?"

"We gave the family two hundred pounds of millet as a settlement."

I never heard anything about him again, but I thought of him often throughout my life, wondering what became of him. The soldier made a deep impression on me.

There was another patient who left a deep impression on me during the war. His surname was Li, the same as mine. He was carried into the clinic on a stretcher with his face downward because his butt had been injured by machine-gun shots. He had to lie flat on his stomach with his butt facing up all the time. He was ill-tempered, constantly swatting the nurses with a walking stick. As a result, no one wanted to go near to him. Because I was new, they gave me the job of taking care of him. Every time I went to change the dressing on his wounded behind, he hit me with his walking stick for no reason. Finally, I got angry and didn't change his dressing for four days. On the morning of the fifth day, I heard him shouting and cursing. I opened the bandage and found maggots in the wound. The head nurse was furious when she found out.

"How could you do that? You will be held responsible if he dies," she yelled.

"But he hit me with a stick every time I got near him. You can ask anyone if you don't believe me," I said.

"There is no excuse for your behavior," she said.

I was criticized — and scared to death. I couldn't imagine what would happen if the patient died of infection or something else. Not only did the patient live but, to my surprise, his wound healed much faster than it normally would have, and in two weeks he was back on the battlefield. It was a miracle. We figured that the worms ate away the rotten tissue, allowing the wound to recover much quicker. In the next meeting, I was praised for the invention of "worm treatment," which was soon introduced to other medical teams within the division.

At the time, Chiang Kai-shek's Nationalists were fleeing south. Rumor had it that in some cases they burned all the grain that they couldn't take with them to prevent it from falling into the hands of the Communist troops. Even with financial support from the U.S., the Nationalists were still crippled by rampant corruption within the government and enormous debt. They paid off these debts by printing more money, causing hyperinflation. It was said that inflation was so bad that the same amount of money that could buy an ox in the beginning of the Nationalists' regime, could only purchase a few grains of rice in the end. Around this time, the 13th Brigade had been organized into the Fourth Field Army directed by Lin Biao, who later became the country's vice-chairman. The Eighth Route Army was redesigned as the People's Liberation Army.

When we reached Shanhaiguan Pass, the so-called "first pass under heaven," the troop was held up for three months, fighting back and forth with the Nationalists. I had a chance to visit the temple of Meng Jiangnu, several miles east of the pass. According to legend, Meng Jiangnu traveled a long distance from Shanxi to bring winter clothes to her husband, who was enslaved at Shanhaiguan Pass to build the Great Wall for Emperor Qin. Learning that he had died while performing hard labor, she sobbed for seven days and nights, until the Great Wall collapsed along a stretch of hundreds of miles, revealing the bones of her husband.

I was given the task of caring for seven wounded soldiers. This time the ward was set up in an old woman's home in a village, where I treated the patients, and, at the same time, cooked and washed clothes for them. After returning to the troop with the seven recovered soldiers, I was awarded a third-class merit citation for taking such good care of the patients. The certificate of merit was handwritten and the paper was lost a long time ago, but the event was recorded in my personal file, which the party kept.

It was at this time that I developed a severe stomach pain and extremely high fever, which made it difficult for me to walk. To ease the pain, I was given a bottle of opium to drink. I grabbed the bottle, desperately gulped down a large amount and became overdosed. I began vomiting and my entire body was itchy. A doctor diagnosed the problem as appendicitis, which required surgery. They transferred me to the Fourth Medical Unit of Jidong Military Region in Hebei Province.

The hospital was stationed in a small village. After my surgery, the incision became infected. The hospital leader reluctantly gave permission to use antibiotics, which were in short supply. Shortly after the injection of the antibiotics, I started noticing mild spasms in my jaw, face, and neck area; they rapidly developed in my chest, back, and abdomen, and eventually spread throughout my whole body. It turned out that the needle a nurse had injected me with had been previously used on a tetanus patient and was not disinfected. I contracted tetanus, which was more deadly than my original infection. When the seizure suddenly attacked, my entire body twitched uncontrollably in anguish as I clenched my teeth.

When they transferred me to a special ward for tetanus patients, even with my limited medical knowledge, I figured out that the death rate for tetanus was two out of three. There were eight patients in the beginning but that number dwindled as the dead were carried out each day. They had left me there to die. I gave all my belongings to the nurse who was taking care of me. "Keep the things you like and hand over to the army the things you don't want," I said to her.

"I'm dying," I said to the doctor who came to the ward to check on me.

"You are just paranoid. It's not that serious," he said to me. I knew in my heart that he was saying something that he himself didn't even believe.

After the doctor left, two dogs began fighting furiously in the yard, which caused me to become agitated and flip into a convulsion. "This is it!" I said to myself. I envisioned the demons with ropes in their hands coming to escort me away.

The nurse grabbed me and cried hysterically. I didn't realize that such a close relationship had developed between us during my short stay in the hospital. I wanted to tell her to go get a doctor at once, but I couldn't open my mouth to speak due to the lockjaw, and she just kept crying. After the seizure was over, a sense of calm came over me. I wasn't sure whether I was dead or alive. When I finally opened my eyes, the nurse told me I had been sleeping for two days. I looked around the ward. I was the only patient left.

I spent three months in the hospital ward. After recovering, I wanted to go back to the army where I belonged. The hospital leader persuaded me to stay and work for them, since he knew I was a medic. "You can make the revolution anywhere. We need medical staff anyway, so why not just stay here? Besides, your 13th Brigade is faraway south now. How could you hope to catch up with them?" he said to me. I thought that sounded reasonable and agreed to stay. But I didn't want to work in the Fourth Medical Unit where I had almost died.

After the ordeal, my medical knowledge increased substantially. The old proverb made sense, I thought to myself. "You become an excellent doctor after breaking your collarbone three times."

5

Love and War

In May of 1949, Chiang Kai-shek fled to Taiwan. In September, I was transferred to the 201 Division headquarters in Changli, Hebei Province, to work in a clinic. Less than a month later, Chairman Mao declared the establishment of the People's Republic of China. On that day, we were issued new green-colored uniforms and the whole division of soldiers gathered in the exercise ground to celebrate the important event. We didn't know exactly what was going on in Beijing because nobody had a radio at the time. So we listened to the officials' speeches and watched the shows that the soldiers themselves had put on including the Shandong clapper ballad and crosstalk, a form of stand-up comedy where two comedians perform together. In the middle of it, a sudden downpour put a damper on the celebration. My new uniform was soaked through and I was shivering with cold. Soon the assembly was dismissed and I ran quickly into the dorm to change clothes.

Many years later, I had the chance to see the historical event of the founding ceremony in a documentary movie. Mao's voice was shaky due to the low quality of the aged film. "The Chinese people have stood up," Chairman Mao declared in his Hunan accent, indicating the Chinese were freed from the "three big mountains" — imperialism, feudalism, and bureaucrat-capitalism, which weighed heavily on their backs before liberation. He gave the speech on the rostrum of

Tiananmen while hundreds of thousands of people below cheered and shouted, "Long live Chairman Mao."

In the chairman's speech he also stated the creation of "people's democratic dictatorship," which was soon put into practice. In March 1950, the party issued its "directive on resolute suppression of counter-revolutionaries" to wipe out the enemies of the state, actual and potential. In a few short years, millions of landlords, rich merchants, and criminals were executed after hasty mass trials attended by thousands of people. The violent campaign reached its peak in 1951. Since there was no criminal law or civil code under Mao's rule, arbitrary procedures were the only way to handle trials. During this time, the army also screened the soldiers for political problems. A nurse in my clinic was found to have a questionable political background. Her father was a landlord before liberation and was executed during the campaign of "suppression of the counter-revolutionaries." Even though she was very diligent in her work, she still couldn't earn the party's trust. There was another female soldier who also had a problem because her fiancé had run away with the Nationalists to Taiwan.

In the beginning of 1950, an order was issued to demobilize a certain percentage of soldiers to relieve the burden on the country. China was one of the most destitute countries in the world. In the countryside the peasants, who comprised more than eighty percent of the population, exploited by landlords and vulnerable to frequent natural disasters like flood, drought, and locust plagues, lived on the edge of starvation. Throughout history, famine periodically reduced the population by millions. Killer diseases such as plague, cholera, and smallpox (respectively referred to in China as "No. 1, No. 2 and No. 3 diseases") were prevalent, while few people had access to doctors. The cities were ravaged by massive unemployment, corruption, skyrocketing inflation, opium addiction, and prostitution. Eighty percent of the people were illiterate because they couldn't afford even a basic education.

With eight years of the Anti-Japanese War and four years of the Civil War behind them, most soldiers had become accustomed to army life and were reluctant to leave, especially those from the countryside, who weren't looking forward to becoming peasants again. The political department put significant effort into persuading the frustrated soldiers. "You came for the sake of revolution, and you shall leave for the sake of revolution," they said. They didn't know that in the very near future they would have to reverse all of their hard work and coax the soldiers to stay.

There were a great number of officers who were getting to be thirty or forty years old and still remained single. Now that the Civil War was over, it was a good time to get married and have families. Some married officers, many of whose marriages had been arranged by their parents before they joined the army, divorced their wives and married younger women.

Many officers found wives wherever the troop was stationed. The local girls admired them and were willing to marry officers who were twenty or thirty years their senior. In particular, the pretty actresses from the cultural troupe were in great demand. For those officers who had difficulty finding a partner, the party officials would step in to arrange a match for them just as their parents would have done.

Colleagues tried to match me up with several older and illiterate officers, each of whom was old enough to be my father. I never agreed. One of the old officials was Commissar Feng, but I didn't have any romantic feelings toward him, though I did respect him.

A day before the Moon Festival, lunar August 15, an officer in the supply department approached me.

"I want you to meet someone," he said.

"I don't want to know anyone," I said, afraid that he was going to suggest one of those old men.

Seeming to know what I was thinking, he said, "Don't worry. I don't want to find you an old man."

"Who is he?" I was curious.

"His name is Han Wende. He is the accountant in the finance section."

"How old is he?" I asked. The fact that he might be both young and an official seemed too good to be true.

"Twenty-five."

"We are the same age," I said, thinking that his age was perfect. "What does he look like?" I asked. I didn't want to marry someone ugly either.

"Very handsome," he said firmly. "Why don't I arrange for you to meet and you can see for yourself?"

I couldn't believe my luck. He was young and handsome, not to mention that he was also a company commander, a fairly high rank for his age. From what the matchmaker kept telling me, I didn't think it sounded too bad at all, but I didn't want to be formally introduced until I'd seen him first. I would feel awkward if it didn't work out, and I also didn't want to appear too eager. Besides, dating wasn't so open those days.

"How should we meet?" I asked the matchmaker.

"At lunchtime, watch who I will hit. That will be him. Observe from the side," he said.

I had heard of many different ways that a matchmaker got people together, but it was the first time I had heard of introducing someone by hitting him. A strange way to introduce someone, but it got to the point. At first all I wanted was to see what the person looked like. And that was how I met my husband.

At noon, Wende showed up in the canteen wearing a white shirt, swinging a lunch box casually in his hand, completely unaware of what was going on. The matchmaker suddenly came up behind him, slapping him firmly on the back three times while I stood watching nearby. Actually, I had laid eyes on Wende before but had never had an opportunity to talk to him. He was a very good-looking man with a face that was honest and kind, almost childish. Since he was completely in the dark about the whole plot, I could observe him at close range without any embarrassment.

The next day, the Moon Festival, which was traditionally celebrated by eating moon cakes, Wende and I were formally introduced to each other. We were invited to the matchmaker's home and had a pleasant meal, followed by moon cakes and some delicious oversized grapes, well known throughout Hebei Province. After the meal, we were left alone so we could chat in private.

We turned out to be the perfect match and were quite happy with each other, which filled all of the old officers, especially Commissar Feng, with jealousy. Just like the matchmaker said, Wende was young and handsome, and he talked in a slow and gentle tone. I really couldn't find much wrong with him except for the fact that he was a noisy eater, which I assumed was a bad habit that he would break after we got married. But he never did. He maintained the habit his whole life. I don't know why such a trivial thing bothered me so much.

On a Sunday in 1950, after we had known each other for about eight months, I walked the three miles from the hospital to the supply department to visit Wende. We went to a photo studio in town to have our first picture taken together. Wende's mother, who lived in the countryside in Hebei Province, had requested a picture of me, her future daughter-in-law.

Even though everything seemed to be going well, our romance was overshadowed by the self-serving intent of the matchmaker, and the war cloud that hung over the Korean Peninsula.

In the fall of 1950, four months after the Korean War broke out, I went on a trip to the provinces of Shanxi, Sichuan, and Anhui to recruit new soldiers for the troop. The political task of demobilizing soldiers had to be reversed. Not only did they have to persuade the soldiers to stay, but they needed more soldiers.

At that time, Shanxi was a very poor place where all the villagers lived in caves. It is located on the world's largest loess plateau, where the Yellow River passes through, carrying mud and sand that turn the water into a yellow color. It is difficult for trees to survive because the impoverished dusty yellow earth is vulnerable to the forces of wind and rain. Loss of soil during the rainy summer season is a serious problem.

For thousands of years, the cave dwellings were built by carving into the loess soil in the region. The fronts of the caves all face south to take in the sunshine. We stayed with one family who had been living in the cave for many generations. Strings of red pepper and corn hung down from the eaves, a typical scene in the area. When I first entered the cave, I saw several baskets of potatoes on the adobe kitchen counter and later found out that those were our supper. Potatoes were their principal food. That was all we ate during the several days we stayed. The host boiled a big pot of them and we gathered around a short table on the adobe *kong* bed with our legs crossed to eat in the bean-oil-lamp-lit cave. The cave was very warm and cozy on those cold days. Even today, there are about 40 million people who still live in the cave dwellings spread all over the region.

Anhui was one of the destitute provinces lying on the traditional famine belt between the two major rivers: Yellow River and Yangtze River. The founder of the Ming dynasty, Zhu Yuanzhang, a beggar who became the emperor, was from Anhui Province. Many country boys there were willing to join the army in order to get away from the hard life in the countryside. We recruited a couple of thousand soldiers on the tour. Those southerners are quite small, fair-skinned, and very soft-spoken, quite different from the northerners. The soldiers from Sichuan liked to eat hot peppery food and rice.

At midnight, a few days after the new recruits arrived, the bugle resonated throughout the chilly night air. It was an emergency muster. Soldiers responded by getting up immediately.

Each packed all of his belongings, his quilt and food, into one knapsack. Then they all headed to a predetermined meeting spot, within fifteen minutes. Since I had practiced the procedure diligently, I was able to complete the whole drill in only five minutes. My knapsack looked neat and orderly upon my back, and, of course, I was one of the first to arrive at the muster spot. The new soldiers who had just been recruited could never get the exercise done in fifteen minutes. They had never been through what I had. I could hear them yelling in all kinds of different accents and dialects.

"Why do we always come out at night like a bunch of rats?" a soldier from Anhui complained. He was short, thin, and pale with a very feminine demeanor. He came out of the camp carrying a quilt and shoes in his arms. After the troop assembled, we set out on a march of up to fifty miles.

A week after I came back from the recruitment trip, I met Wende again and he had a gift for me: a beautiful watch.

"You shouldn't have spent so much money," I said.

"No, I didn't buy it. It's from our matchmaker," he told me.

"Why did he give you such an expensive gift?"

"He was just trying to be nice. He told me I could pay him back later. He said, 'You two have known each other for several months now. The military exercises have started and no one knows what is going to happen. If you are sent to Korea and she stays here, there could be a problem. A long delay means trouble. She's getting older and may not wait for you.' He thought we should write an application for approval to get married."

"But that doesn't explain the watch. Besides, how does he know I won't wait for you?"

"If you agree, let's write a marriage application," Wende said. I knew it was something he had thought about for a long time; it was not just a spur of the moment decision. So I agreed.

When the troop moved north to Jinxi, now Huludao City, Wende wrote an application for approval of our marriage and handed it in. The person who reviewed the marriage application was Commissar Feng. Our request was denied, and the reason given was: "The male has not reached the stipulated age. Marriage is not permitted. However, you have permission to maintain your relationship." I suspected that the refusal might have had something to do with Commissar Feng's personal feelings.

"You have reached the stipulated age; I haven't. I don't want to hold you up. If you find anyone suitable, just forget about me," Wende said to me, the disappointment clearly showing on his face, even though he tried to conceal it.

"It's not a big deal. I'll wait for you for a couple of more years," I said.

"You mean that?"

"Of course I do."

"Okay, don't blame me if you get too old and nobody wants to marry you," he joked.

After that, we couldn't see each other in private anymore — a necessity if we were to avoid harmful gossip. We looked forward to every Saturday because this was the one day that all units in the division got together to exercise. We would both open our eyes wide looking for each other in the sea of soldiers in the exercise grounds. It was not an easy task to find a person in a whole infantry division of thousands of soldiers running around dressed in the same uniform. In fact, everyone looked so alike, that, from a distance, it was even a challenge to tell a male and female apart. After spotting each other, we would just smile with understanding, which was better than a thousand words. We waited a whole week just to give each other a smile.

It didn't take long for us to realize that the reason the officer was so eager to be the matchmaker wasn't just to be neighborly, but to use Wende's position as the accountant of the finance section to help him embezzle funds. In fact, it turned out that there were several other people, including a fairly high-ranking official, involved in the plan to win Wende over, but he was an honest man and couldn't be persuaded to join the gang.

"Valiantly and Spiritedly,
I Fell into the Yalu River"

On the freezing night of March 8, 1951, cooks in the kitchen squad began a flatbread-making campaign, suddenly preparing great amounts of this particular starchy food for the whole 201 Division. It was unclear to everyone why so much flatbread had to be made. Even the cooks themselves were kept in the dark. After the flatbread was done, it was distributed among the soldiers, who put their shares into big, white food bags.

At nine-thirty, the bugle blared, announcing the emergency muster. With heavy confused steps, the soldiers raced to the assembly place with knapsacks on their backs. When the troop set out to the railway station, Wende came to see me off.

"I was appointed as a platoon commander just a minute ago. There are eighteen paramedics under my command," I said to him. "They are all new recruits. They don't seem to be able to get used to the hard life in the army."

"So where are you heading?" he asked.

"I don't know. We are not allowed to talk about it. I don't even know why we have to carry so much flatbread, it's so heavy," I said, and threw some of it away when no one was looking.

We also had to carry five pounds of peanuts, two pounds of salt, four pounds of rice, and two bulky Soviet-made grenades. Platoon commanders and those above this rank were given handguns. Soldiers were divided into groups of three; each group was allowed a rifle or machine gun, which we took turns carrying. In addition to that, the medical teams had to haul supplies: medicine, equipment, and bandages. We needed to be prepared to treat at least two hundred soldiers at any time or place without reinforcement from the supply department. The pale, undersized soldier from Anhui was so small that the weight of his knapsack exceeded his own body weight.

"So when is your department leaving?" I asked Wende.

"Several days after you," he said with a lost expression on his face.

"We'll be seeing each other in a few days then," I said.

"I have a photo of myself for you as a keepsake. I cut the bottom of the photo off," he said. Since this mission was highly secretive, the bottom of his photo, which displayed the "Chinese People's Liberation Army," had to be cut off.

"I don't have anything to give you. Here's a pen. Something to remind you of me," I said.

The army boarded a cargo train with only a vent on the top. The train didn't have any windows at all, which meant we couldn't tell the direction in which we were heading. Since there were no seats, soldiers sat on the floor, side by side. When the mighty steam engine rumbled to life, with tons of metal thrusting forward on the narrow steel track, it let out a piercing shriek that humbled my feelings of sentimentality, making them seem so insignificant at that moment. At first I was restless and nervous. Later the monotonous rumble of the train caused me to doze off with a rifle in my arms.

Hours later, the train came to a halt beside a small station. Light filtered through a gap in the train wall. I stepped off the train onto solid ground. It was a wonderful sensation to stand and stretch in the cold refreshing air.

"Andong station," a soldier with a Sichuan accent said.

"Where is Andong?" came a funny Shanxi tone.

"Here's Andong."

I could hear the whisper of disoriented soldiers as they tried to figure out where they were. They were too worn out to come up with any logical answers, so the conversation soon dwindled. Andong, now known as Dandong, was a small city situated at the Chinese and North Korean border. The city around us lay in darkness and the civilians slept soundly in the silent city, totally unaware of what was going on. To the troops, however, the situation was about to become crystal clear: Commissar Feng began a motivational speech to pump up the soldiers before battle.

"The American imperialists have invaded Korea. They are massacring Korean people and intend to invade China. In order to defend our motherland and ensure world peace, we Chinese volunteers are going to fight in Korea to support the Korean people and beat the American imperialists," he declared.

Our 201 Division wasn't the first Chinese troop entering Korea. Major troops entered Korea in October 1950. Some said it was as early as July, a month after the Korean War broke out. The Korean War began in the predawn hours of June 25, 1950, when North Korean troops invaded South Korea by crossing the 38th parallel that divided the two countries. The UN swiftly declared war on the North. Initially, North Koreans advanced at an amazing speed, taking Seoul, the capital, in a mere three days, seizing most of the country except for the Pusan perimeter — a small area in the most southeastern corner of the peninsula where the UN troops were forced to retreat. However, the tables turned suddenly when the American General MacArthur, commander of the UN force, staged his daring and brilliant Inchon landing that cut the already overextended North Korean's supply lines and shattered them. By November, UN forces had already reached the Yalu River and Kim's Communist regime was nearly wiped off the map.

However, the situation changed abruptly after Chairman Mao decided to help out his defeated Communist neighbor with limited assistance from the Soviet Union. He feared that UN troops would cross the Yalu River and "strangle the one-year-old new Communist China in its cradle." At least that was what we were told. The real motive for Mao sending troops is still unknown, and it continues to be a subject under debate. Some speculate that Stalin used the Chinese as cannon fodder during the Cold War, while others think that he didn't mastermind the Chinese involvement, but that it was Mao who took advantage of the situation to either teach the Americans a lesson or to use it as a bargaining tool to pressure the Soviets to arm China. During that time, China massed 850,000 troops north of the river. The Chinese troops rapidly pushed toward the south, crossing the 38th parallel, throwing the UN forces back midway into South Korea. However, the Chinese were primitively equipped with rifles that were mostly captured from the Japanese and Nationalists during the wars, and could only go on offensive operations that lasted no more than a week, at which point a pause was required for new supplies — often delayed due to air raids. Attacking and counterattacking, the war soon phased into a stalemate, neither side achieving a decisive victory. Truce talks began in July 1951, but the fighting didn't stop until two years later.

The Chinese called the conflict "The War to Resist America and Aid Korea." Our army was referred to as "volunteer troops," which coincidentally had a very similar pronunciation to "aiding troops." Since nobody had really volunteered, I just thought in terms of "aiding troops" without ever truly understanding the original meaning of the words. The reason the troop was given the name "volunteers" was that Mao didn't want to give the impression that China had declared war with the U.S. and risk escalating the war.

Shortly before our troop set out, I heard a gunshot echo through the quiet night. A literacy instructor had injured his hand. I was called to assist the surgeon who would perform the surgery. During the operation the instructor tearfully confessed the truth. He had deliberately shot himself because he was afraid to go to Korea. In an attempt to make it appear an accident, he had fired at his right hand with a Russian-made handgun, thinking it would only create a small hole — enough to get himself discharged from duty. To his surprise, however, the bullet exploded when it encountered blood and his whole hand had to be amputated.

"Intellectuals! We've got to keep an eye on them," Commissar Feng said to me.

When the Yalu River appeared in front of me out of nowhere, and brought a cold wet breeze to my face, the tiredness of the train ride slipped away. My heart started beating so wildly that I was certain the soldier beside me could hear the loud thumping in the silence of the night. When I glanced back at the city, it was bathed in complete darkness. The Yalu River was dark and appeared motionless. It was impossible to make out which direction the water was flowing.

Before I could make sense of it all, I was already on the bridge to North Korea. The heavy steps of the soldiers, who were carrying backpacks and guns, along with the labored breathing of the mules and horses weighted down with ammunition, blended together, becoming chaotic. Our troop wore nothing on our uniforms to indicate who we were, and we formed a shadowy mass making its way toward the other end of the bridge. In the middle of the bridge, a white line had been drawn representing the border between China and Korea. It was just a single line, but when I stepped over it, a strange feeling suddenly overcame me. I was in a foreign country now.

I heard frantic voices calling out. "Someone fell into the river!"

In the turmoil — with the troops, mules, and horses sharing the crowded narrow bridge — the soldier from Anhui had been squeezed to the bridge edge, lost his balance, and plunged into the dark Yalu River below. After he was saved, he created his own version of the people's volunteer army battle song. Instead of "Valiantly and spiritedly, we cross the Yalu River. To defend peace and our county, our motherland," he sang: "Valiantly and spiritedly, I fell into the Yalu River. . . ."

★

"Chinese soldiers and officers!" a strange voice rang out the next morning.

The soldiers heard an American broadcast being amplified from an airplane with a loudspeaker. The announcer was Chinese. "I am a Chinese. I graduated from Beijing University. Don't be afraid. This is not a bomber. There is only a pilot and myself in the plane. The pilot doesn't speak Chinese so I am his assistant. We are a UN peacekeeping force. The North Korean Army has invaded South Korea. . . . Your 201 Division with backward weapons cannot win the war. Soldiers! Go back to where you came from. . . ."

"How the hell do they know we are the 201 Division?" The soldiers were puzzled.

The soldiers gave the U.S. aircraft many nicknames. They called the scouting plane *The Hanging Ghost*. It was a strange-looking thing that hovered in the air like someone hanging. If it stayed in one area for a long time, this usually meant that it had found something suspicious. As soon as it was out of sight, the *Big Claws* — a large fleet of twenty or thirty bombers — would arrive and start a massive assault with bombs, napalm, and machine-gun-strikes, all at the same time, just like eagles seizing their prey.

During the Korean War, the Chinese troops didn't have any anti-aircraft weapons, so scouting planes and the bombers could do as much damage as possible and the soldiers were just like a piece of meat on a cutting board. There was an order issued from above that prohibited soldiers from trying to shoot down scouting planes with light arms like rifles because, if they failed, the troop's position would be exposed to the enemy.

To avoid air raids, the troop marched at night and by day rested in the forest. Even at night the safety of the troop wasn't guaranteed because the enemy detonated illuminating shells. These were so powerful that they could light up an entire area within a one-mile radius, their luminescence appearing much brighter against the silvery snow. We had to stop each time an illuminating shell was lit up and continue after it went off. Strong searchlights were also employed, which could throw out a far-reaching beam of light to scan the perimeter for any activity. The enemy often created a blockade of intermittent crossfire to prevent Chinese troops from passing a crucial location. With every step, the soldiers faced imminent danger.

Being from Inner Mongolia, I was acquainted with harsh weather. Still, the excruciating cold and the long march made my knees feel as though they were being poked by needles. A few months earlier, the first troops had entered Korea in such a hasty manner that the Chinese soldiers from the south were without winter coats and boots, leaving them totally unprepared for such severe weather. The temperature fell dramatically to forty below zero, taking soldiers by surprise. Many soldiers suffered from third-degree frostbite which caused their outer skin and the underneath tissue to become severely damaged, resulting in gangrene that required amputation. Some got it so bad that their feet and shoes froze together into one painful mass. Overnight, there were soldiers frozen to death. They had to bury them in the shallow snow because the ground was frozen so solid that it was impossible to dig holes into it.

As we continued to advance south, the soldiers ate their bland diet of parched flour mixed with snow. It wasn't very appealing, but at least it was food. The parched flour was dropped from Chinese transport planes in big pails. Since they had no way to pinpoint the exact position of the troops, quite often they missed us by miles. On the third week, we reached Pyongyang, the North Korean capital, only to discover that it had been almost completely demolished and corpses littered the ground. A dead mother, wearing a blood-tinted white blouse and short vest, had been lying in the ruins with her small infant still sucking innocently on her nipple. The baby was sent to an orphanage in China, the place where many children without parents ended up during the war. After witnessing the horrors of Pyongyang, we forged ahead to the south.

After a few days' march, we arrived at an airport. However, there was no plane parked there. The runways were seriously damaged by bombing. We stayed there for two weeks to repair them. During the Korean War, China didn't have many planes and the government called on citizens to donate money to buy some.

The snow turned into springtime rain. Liberated from our bulky winter clothes, we moved more quickly through the rugged mountains and headed toward the 38th parallel. As we climbed through the slippery mountain passes, for support we had to catch hold of the end of each other's raincoats, which were made of waterproof oilcloth. If anyone released his grip, he could plunge to his death off the steep cliff.

Initially, when we drank the water from the mountain streams, we added a few water purification drops, but over time, we became accustomed to its sweet taste and didn't bother to add any drops.

Occasionally, if luck was on our side, we would find a house in the village to lodge in, but most of the time we set up camp in the forest by utilizing two pieces of oilcloth, one to construct a tent and the other one for bedding. Three soldiers formed a small group, each taking turns being on guard while the other two slept. Plenty of snakes slithered through the campsite. I had been quite content sleeping on the oilcloth, with thick comfortable leaves beneath it until one morning when we took down the tent and I discovered, to my horror, that there had been a huge snake under the oilcloth the whole time I had slept.

One night we hiked almost a hundred miles. Everyone was so exhausted that we looked forward to the dawn when we could get off our feet and rest. Some soldiers became so tired that they fell asleep while marching. As the first blush of dawn approached, the troop was crossing the Qingjiang Bridge. The soldier from Anhui was almost collapsing from fatigue and refused to walk even one more step, because his feet were in such poor condition that one squeeze of his swollen toes would cause blood and pus to come oozing out. Sitting on the bridge, the thin fair-skinned soldier appeared quite fragile in his baggy uniform.

"The bridge is not a safe place to rest," I said to him. "We have come all this way so you can't quit now. When we cross the bridge you can rest."

"No, I can't walk anymore. Every step I take is like walking on nails," he said.

"It's close to dawn. The U.S. bombers may come at any time. You have to get up and move!"

"I don't care. I might as well let them kill me and get it over with."

"If you won't walk, then you will have to crawl," I said. I removed his rifle and dragged him all the way across the bridge, using strength that I didn't even know I had. Once across, he joined a special unit that cared for those who fell behind.

Shortly after we crossed the bridge, a cluster of U.S. bombers arrived on the scene, dropped numerous bombs on the bridge, completely destroying it. Wende's supply department was cut off from my troop on the other side of the bridge — which meant our food and supplies were also cut off.

For twenty-five torturous days, the only food our empty stomachs saw was parched flour, and when that eventually ran out, soldiers hurried to the fields to collect wild vegetables. As the rain poured down, I led six nurses on a search for edible weeds using a little book about wild vegetables that the Koreans had given us for reference.

After a month of hardship, against all odds Wende's department finally caught up with us and replenished our food and medical supplies. We met the evening before we had to set out again. We relaxed for a moment under a big chestnut tree.

"We all ran out of food and medical supplies. I don't know what would have happened if you hadn't shown up," I said.

"We managed to cross the river after the bridge was blown up during the air strike. We had to travel at night to avoid air raids and drivers were not allowed to use headlights, so several trucks fell over the cliff. It could be also because they had to drive straight through the long night and became overly tired," he reported.

Dusk was all around us, the sunset turning the sky into a glowing spectacle of red and orange. Birds were returning to their nests, twittering in the big chestnut tree. It was a beautiful evening and, for a moment, I forgot that I was in a battlefield in a foreign country faraway from home.

"I hope this will all be over soon so we can go home, and get married, and have a family," Wende said in his usual slow tone.

"It's funny that before we crossed the Yalu River, Commissar Feng told us to prepare ourselves for three months in Korea. After crossing the river, he suddenly changed his tone and told us to get ready for a protracted war. Who knows how long we are going to be here," I said.

"What time are you setting out?" he asked me.

"At seven tonight. And you?"

"At nine."

"Why so late?"

"The darker the better."

I heard the sound of cranking engines as, one by one, the trucks were started and began moving. Birds flew away chirping. We were supposed to leave after dark, but for some unknown reason, Commissar Feng had changed the schedule and ordered us to leave now.

Suddenly came the deafening roar of bombers as they tore through the sky above us. When I looked up, about thirty bombers were already upon us. They flew so low that I could even make out the symbols on the aircrafts. The soldiers were stunned. Without an order, no one dared to make a move. Finally we heard the commissar's voice.

"I order everyone to get off the road and take cover!"

Soldiers sprung off the trucks and scattered in all directions.

The sky suddenly darkened when an explosion of napalm, fire, smoke, whistling shrapnel, machine-gun strikes, flying rocks and dust, and the blood-curdling shrieks of soldiers all mingled together. An inferno erupted around us, devouring the mountain and forest with its flames. Napalm bombs, containing jellied gasoline, could turn an area the size of a football field into a sea of fire. The chemical substance sticks to anything it touches and burns at a temperature of 3,000 degrees Celsius. It causes agonizing pain and suffering. Another lethal property is that it sucks oxygen out of the air, and produces carbon monoxide which leads to suffocation. It was said that more napalm was dropped during the three-year Korean War than during the prolonged Vietnam War. When such a bomb was dropped over a forest, the inferno would be ablaze for days. The ear-splitting sound of the constant explosions echoed in the mountains. It was so intense I felt as though someone was hammering my heart and that it was unable to withstand the shock.

Wende caught on fire. He rolled on the ground while I tried to extinguish the flames with a tree branch. Suddenly bullets peppered the ground right beside us, stirring the thick dust. Seconds later, bullets struck again from the other direction, this time even closer.

"That was close!" I said to Wende later.

"We are so lucky to be alive," he said and sighed with relief.

After the bombers left, just as quickly as they had arrived, the shell-shocked troop reassembled. It didn't take long to assess the number of casualties. All the injured soldiers were transferred to a hospital that was hastily set up in an old abandoned mine, which was located in a deep valley surrounded by mountains. All the trucks and supplies had been destroyed.

"The food is here." At supper time, the cook carried food trays directly into the operating rooms. I ate with surgical clothing on, and after finishing, I put my mask and gloves back on and continued working. When the large-scale battles got underway, the casualties poured in. It was the sixth straight day and night that I had worked without rest. Even though the Chinese troops succeeded in their surprise attack on the UN troops at the end of 1950, by early 1951 we were at the end of our logistics supply line. The Americans staged Operation Killer in February and Operation Ripper in March. In spring, they pushed across the 38th parallel for the second time. During this period, the Chinese troops suffered extremely heavy casualties — often whole battalions of soldiers would vanish. In one case, the entire 180 Division of 60 Army was completely wiped out.

With my three-month crash course in battlefield surgery, I became an assistant to a surgeon who was performing major operations. The surgeon was considered the best in the division and was appropriately nicknamed the "First Knife of 201 Division." There were several operating rooms and they were all busy. It was like hell on earth with the sickly odor of blood, the shouts of medics with different accents, and the moaning of patients in extreme anguish.

"Copper saw." The surgeon extended his hand, but nothing happened.

He raised his voice. "Hand me the copper saw."

Since the surgeon hadn't asked for a tool in a while, I had dozed off while carrying a surgical tool tray.

I woke up and handed him a small copper saw and heard the usual, chilling sound of the instrument cutting through bone. The soldier let out blood-curdling screams of agony. Since there was a great shortage of anesthetic and only the officials were entitled to use it, the average soldiers called it "cadre's medicine." As an assistant, my job was also to do "ideological work" for the patients before, during, and after the surgery. Before the surgery, I had to explain why the amputation was necessary. The worst part of the job was during the surgery when I had to tell the patients to be strong and not to cry out even though I knew that they were enduring great pain. In preparing for the amputation, I would tie the patient firmly to the operating table with belts to prevent him from struggling, then spray the wounded area with saltwater to prevent infection. After the limb was severed, the surgeon would tie up the major arteries and sew up the skin with catgut — a cord made from the dried intestines of sheep or other animals. This kind of stitch would be absorbed by the body over time. Because of the lack of medicine and poor sanitation, it was common for patients to die from infection after surgery. The surgeon tossed the severed bloody arm, still twitching, into the enormous pile of dismembered limbs in the corner of the operating room. At nightfall, I disposed of the countless arms and legs by burying them in a hole outside at the back of the operating rooms. I could hear the blast of bombs exploding in the distance and saw them light up the silhouette of the mountains. The fury of the bombs and guns would intensify at times, but occasionally it would quiet down and the night would become almost tranquil.

After burying the limbs, it would be time for me to make my round of the ward, which sheltered over two hundred patients. The interior was permeated with the foul stench of human waste that covered the soldiers' uniforms. Since they had no choice but to use the trenches as bathrooms, when the battle got underway they would end up rolling around in their own excrement. The ward was made up of two rows of beds with a corridor running through the middle. Patients lay side by side, calling out in agony for medicine to ease their pain. I tied the bottom of my pants with string so lice and fleas wouldn't crawl up.

Patients suffering from second- and third-degree burns were common. These patients experienced extreme pain, except for one patient who didn't feel anything because third-degree burns had covered eighty-five percent of his body surface and destroyed all of the nerves.

A captured American pilot was among the patients. As soon as he saw me, he took out the little book that every captive carried in their pockets and showed me. It was about the UN's policy concerning the treatment of POWs printed in English, Chinese, and Korean. Then he showed me the picture of his wife and son. The pilot had injured one of his feet, and was trying to make me understand that he was in pain by gesturing to his foot, and repeatedly saying, "trouble, trouble" in English. I placed a pillow under his leg to elevate his foot and he soon felt better. The POWs were given the same portion of food as Chinese patients and also treated with the hospital's limited medical supplies.

While the American captives were writing to their wives and families saying, "I love you and miss you very much," the Chinese patients were writing letters to the Communist Party, pledging to "fight till the last drop of blood."

"Nurse, I'm thirsty," a patient called out in a weak voice.

I recognized it as that of the soldier from Anhui. He had cholera and was already severely dehydrated due to massive watery diarrhea; he had also experienced other symptoms, such as rapid pulse and vomiting. During the Korean War, infectious diseases like cholera and typhus resulted in casualties as great as from any battle. He was scheduled to be sent to the base hospital, located several hundred miles north. From there he might have a chance to be transferred back home to China.

When the time came, all the stretchers were in use, so I had to carry him on my back in the transferring process. For no apparent reason this enraged the patient. He insisted that he should be carried on a stretcher.

"Put me down, damn it! And carry me on a stretcher!" he screamed angrily.

"But we ran out of stretchers," I explained to him.

"I don't care. Just get me a goddamn stretcher," he insisted. He was so infuriated that he used his last bit of strength kicking and struggling like a child on my back. Suddenly he stopped his erratic movement and collapsed. We couldn't transfer him anymore, and the doctors did what they could to revive him but failed. The soldier from Anhui had stopped breathing.

At the time, I was suffering from night blindness caused by the lack of vitamins in our diet. Vegetables were hard to come by and most of the time we had to eat parched flour, the most common food, since it was easy to carry and store. It was not unusual to see soldiers struggling to swallow the parched flour without any water. On that particular night, I was ordered to stay behind because I couldn't see my way around in the dark; meanwhile, other hospital staff continued to transfer patients.

I put my fingers on the pulse of the soldier from Anhui. It was a miracle. He still had a pulse. Perhaps he is just in a coma, I thought to myself. We were alone in the dark and the beating of the pulse seemed so loud in the night air. I looked at him but couldn't make out his face. I could hear the chaotic sounds of medics shouting, patients moaning, and motors rumbling as they mixed together with the distant barrage of guns firing and bombs exploding. Gazing up, I could vaguely see the stars twinkling, but when I looked around, I couldn't make out a thing. The soldiers lived life like a bunch of rats. They stayed in their holes during the daytime and came out at night. Now they were swarming all over the mountains. "Someone come to help me carry the damn stretcher!" I heard someone shout in a Sichuan accent.

An hour had passed. The pulse of the soldier from Anhui still remained, loud and clear, although his body seemed to be getting cold and remained still. It finally occurred to me that I had been with a corpse the whole time. The pulse I felt was not his, but my own. The soldier from Anhui had departed the earth forever. I never understood why he insisted on being carried on a stretcher. All I really knew was that he might still be alive if he hadn't kicked and struggled like that. They might even have sent him home to be with his family.

"Valiantly and spiritedly, I fell into the Yalu River . . ." I couldn't rid the voice from my mind. It drove me crazy.

We were always on the move, never staying in one place for more than two months. The patients in serious condition would be transferred to the base hospital. The "base" was just a relative term since during the Korean War there was no difference between the front and the rear. The whole of North Korea was a battlefield, and U.S. bombers could raid anywhere at any time. Whenever we got to a new place, the first thing we'd do was to see if there were any bomb shelters we could use. If there were none available, we would have to build new ones. To construct ward beds, we usually lay logs side by side on the ground, then put dried grass on top of them. Often there was water in the bomb shelter, and we would have to build beds above it. I could hear the water running under my bed at night. The dampness made my arthritis worse. In July, the peace talks began while the war continued.

From early fall and onward, transmitted diseases led to heavy casualties. First came dysentery, a very serious disease caused by contaminated food and water, characterized by severe diarrhea. It could be fatal if the body became dehydrated enough. In winter, the typhoid fever became prevalent. Typhoid fever is also caused by contaminated food and water, and patients often sustained fevers as high as forty degrees Celsius. Relapsing fever, a louse-born disease, is characterized by repeated episodes of fever. Hemorrhagic fever, caused by viruses that were transmitted by rodents, was also found in the hospital. It was then called Korean hemorrhagic fever because it was first recognized by Western medicine during the Korean War. The symptoms include fever, bleeding under the skin, in the internal organs, and from the nose or eyes. Cholera was also among the diseases I saw. It is characterized by severe diarrhea, and transmitted by contaminated food and water. It was not all that easy to identify a disease without a lab test because some of them shared identical symptoms such as fever and diarrhea. But it didn't matter anyway because the medicine to treat them was limited. Most of these illnesses required antibiotics, the "cadre's medicine," which, as I've said, was in extremely short supply.

In February 1952, officials in the hospital held a meeting to inform us that the Americans had started germ warfare in North Korea. They said that the Americans had dropped flies, lice, and rats which carried diseases such as plague, typhoid, and cholera. Samples of the insects were collected, and the Chinese investigation team confirmed that they carried germs. They said that the Americans had started germ warfare as early as 1951. Rumor had it that the flies that were dropped on the snow from planes were still alive at first, then after a while they froze to death. However the Chinese soldiers still caught the diseases because they often ate parched flour with snow when water was not available. We were put on high alert.

Two days after the meeting, I went out for a short walk with three nurses. It was very dangerous to venture outside of bomb shelters because of air raids and artillery shelling. Unlike bombers, artillery shells could hit at any time without warning so there was no way to prepare for them. I had once seen sixty shells all fall out of the blue in a single area. Also because there were spies around, we were not allowed to go out alone. We had to follow the only trail in the deep snow, and, to avoid falling off the cliff, didn't dare to stray. We were warned not to "burn joss sticks" — freeze to death in the deep snow like joss sticks. The nurses and I walked about fifteen minutes — until the trail came to an abrupt end. About five meters ahead of us was an open, flat area covered with a suspicious dark blanket about half the size of a basketball court. It looked very obvious against the white snow. Most of the dark material was spread evenly, but here and there I could see small clusters that didn't spread out. Could these be the germ-carrying insects the Americans had dropped from the air? We were all in a state of shock. A bold male nurse wanted to take a closer look, but I stopped him.

"The leaders have already warned us about this. We'd better be careful," I said to him. Since I held the rank of platoon commander in charge of the paramedics, he listened to me. When we got back, I reported the incident to officials but they didn't seem to be concerned about it.

"That's just a small patch. The large-scale germ warfare is already over," they told me.

I thought it was a little strange that no precautions were taken in this matter. Then again, there were many other immediate threats than this one.

The dark mass I had seen was suspicious, but there was no way I could confirm that it was germ warfare. In February and March, the Chinese and North Korean governments officially charged the U.S. with using biological weapons. The Americans denied the charge, dismissing it as Communist propaganda, and claimed that the Chinese and North Koreans fabricated evidence.

Before I had no doubt about the Chinese government's accusation but I now have second thoughts. Could these transmittable diseases simply have occurred because of poor nutrition, hygiene, and sanitation among the Chinese soldiers? These terrible living conditions were facts. Often a whole battalion of soldiers would be cramped into one bomb shelter, and being inside this tight enclosed space made it easy for diseases to transmit among them. Body lice was common because soldiers' clothes couldn't be washed or changed. Water couldn't be boiled because smoke would reveal the troops' locations. Poor nutrition also made the soldiers vulnerable to these infectious diseases. Besides, most of these diseases already existed at the time in the Northeast of China where the troops passed through. In the fall of 1950, when we were stationed in Jinxi in the Northeast, we were vaccinated for typhoid. This indicated that this disease was prevalent in the area. Surprisingly, when I talked to several of my old comrades about germ warfare, they all took it as matter of fact. However, when I asked them if they had seen it with their own eyes, they all said no.

7

A Bag of Gold

"Comrade Qunying, report to the office!"

I was right in the middle of a messy surgery when they called me. It was March 1952 and the day was shaping up to be a busy one. A soldier had gotten his leg blown off by a bomb so they delivered him back from the frontline with the severed limb extended grimly beside him on the stretcher.

"What are we going to do with this?" I asked the First Knife, holding the separated leg in my hands.

The surgeon shook his head hopelessly, not saying a word, but I instinctively knew what he meant. We had been busy chopping off damaged arms and legs, never attaching the limbs back to the body. The patient watched as the leg he had been standing on just a while earlier was tossed into the pile in the corner of the operating room like a piece of garbage. I reported to the hospital office.

"We have a new job for you," Commissar Feng said to me.

"What new job?" I asked.

"You will know later. You are going back to China." His tone of voice gave me the impression that he didn't want to explain further. I was trained by the army not to ask questions, to just follow orders.

I was not the only one sent back; in fact, there was quite a collection of us. The people who worked in the financial field from the 199, 200, and 201 Divisions of the 67 Army were thrust together into one group called "study group," which was in fact a concentration camp, and sent back to Tangshan City to be "voluntarily" investigated.

Wende came to say goodbye to me the night before I left for the homeland. His supply department was set up several miles away from the hospital.

"Rumor has it that everyone in the group might have some kind of problem," he said.

"I'm in medical service and have nothing to do with finance at all. What problem could I possibly have?" I said.

"I trust the party will clear things up."

"But there's nothing to clear up. Everything is clear. I'm innocent. I'm not worried," I said. Inside, however, my stomach was churning with worry. It must be serious if they're pulling people away from the battlefield, I thought to myself.

Upon arriving back to Tangshan City, an industrial city about one hundred miles from Beijing, my mind was so consumed with worry that I couldn't sleep for several days. We were detained at a military camp where no one could leave without permission. The camp was about five miles away from the city center. It was next to an abandoned steel factory where I went over to once with some colleagues to take a look. The factory had been very lucrative during the Japanese occupation, but when the Japanese surrendered, the cascading metal soon solidified like a piece of history frozen in time. All the machines lay in ruin. A photo of me was taken that year with the factory in the background.

For the first couple of weeks nothing transpired and no accusations were made, although we were all extremely bored by the monotonous daily meetings in which the officials read from newspapers about corruption, waste, and bureaucracy. My insomnia was made worse by a loudspeaker broadcast that started at five o'clock sharp every morning and rattled on nonstop until midnight. It was all about the Three-Anti's campaign against corruption, waste, and bureaucracy, and the

Five-Anti's campaign against bribery, tax evasion, theft of state
property, and so on. Several major events happened in the
middle of the raging Korean War. The 1950–1952 drive of "suppression of counter-revolutionaries" was accompanied by land
reform — redistribution of land and "class struggle" against
landlords — under the Agrarian Reform Law of June 28, 1950.
On top of those, came the Three-Anti's and Five-Anti's campaigns. The number of people purged by this campaign was
estimated to be in the millions.

We were bombarded by propaganda from every source,
such as newspapers, public blackboards, loudspeakers, and
posters. It wasn't long before they set up a number of locked
wooden boxes with narrow slots to be used for collecting
accusation letters throughout the camp. Everyone was
encouraged, anonymously perhaps, to report, criticize,
accuse, and expose each other.

What had I done wrong? My mind went blank and I
couldn't come up with anything that justified this kind of
treatment. Of course I had made plenty of mistakes, but who
hadn't? The more I thought about it, the more mistakes I realized I had made. I found myself missing Wende considerably.
I began to write him letters, although I hadn't received even
one from him.

After I had been in the study group for three weeks, I was
summoned to the office. I had a bad feeling but pretended to
be calm. Commissar Feng looked across his desk when I
stepped in but didn't greet me. He was smoking a cigarette in
his usual chain-smoking style. When one cigarette was almost
finished, he would use it to light another one.

"I have saved a lot of matches this way," he said to me.

"You called me, Commissar Feng?" I said.

"Comrade Qunying, there's a new job for you," Commissar
Feng said. "You are to officially become a member of the tiger-
hunting group."

"What is the tiger-hunting group?" I asked.

I was soon made aware that "tiger hunting" didn't actually mean heading to the forest, gun in tow, to stalk a wild beast. "A tiger is someone who has embezzled public property and your job is to investigate them."

The commissar continued his explanation: "Embezzling one thousand is a tiger, over two thousand is a big tiger."

"But I have never done anything like this," I said.

"Start with your roommate," the commissar said.

"She didn't do anything wrong. I know her quite well."

"Not well enough. Her husband has embezzled properties. We have already discovered that he hid boxes of silk sheets in his hometown. We have evidence that she knew the scheme. But don't tell her anything — we want her to come forward by herself."

Anyway, I was relieved and realized that I was not a target of the revolution at all; on the contrary, I was going to "revolutionize" other people. All the anguish I had endured over that two-week period had been in vain. The tiger-hunting group was composed of Commissar Feng, officials from 201 Division, and a student from Beijing Qinghua University, who was considered very vicious because he often yelled at people.

All the suspects remained under close watch and were not allowed to go anywhere, but I could go in and out of the camp as I pleased. As an investigator, I went on several long distant trips to places in Hebei and Shanxi Provinces. Many times I came back empty-handed. I was given a ten-page plastic-covered red permit that contained information such as age, sex, rank, and military unit. There was also a big seal and writings of "permission to enter and leave freely." There were two fully armed soldiers carrying rifles with shiny bayonets at the gate. Inside the gatehouse, a machine gun was set up on a desk. The first time I approached the gate, I felt very intimidated. After a soldier handed me back the permit, he saluted me. I instantly felt redeemed, above the others. I had regained my confidence. I should never have doubted myself. How could I have belonged to the suspect group? That night I wrote a letter to Wende to tell him that I was assigned a job in the tiger-hunting group and there was no problem at all.

The wooden boxes were jammed full of accusation letters. There appeared to be a multitude of people implicated for wrongdoing. I went here and there, investigating all the suspects on my long list and collecting incriminating evidence against them. By the end of the day, I would be so weary from my day's labor that I would fall asleep almost immediately, which was an experience I hadn't had for a long while.

My roommate had many sleepless nights before a deadline was arranged. The suspects were informed that if they told the truth before midnight, it would be considered a voluntary confession and would be dealt with leniently; however, anything divulged after midnight would be deemed a sign of guilt, and the suspect would be handled with severity. I tried to give my roommate the hint that she should come forward with the matter, but she insisted that she knew nothing. It might have been my guilty conscience — the night before the deadline, I talked in my sleep and revealed the scheme.

A few minutes before the midnight deadline, my roommate woke me up from my sound sleep. "Wake up, Qunying. I have something to tell you," she whispered.

"Why couldn't you tell me tomorrow?" I said.

"Tonight is the deadline. I've got to expose him."

"Expose who?"

"My husband," she said. "And don't pretend you don't know anything about it. I heard what you said in your sleep. You can't keep a secret. I have something to show you."

I heard a soft jingle as she brought out a chain of keys. "These keys are for the boxes my husband has hidden in his hometown. I swear that I don't know what's in the boxes. He let me keep the keys before he went to Korea. It's already midnight. Please go quickly to tell the officials that I have come clean before the deadline," she said.

"I'll tell them tomorrow. Go back to sleep."

"But the deadline is midnight."

"Don't worry. I'll explain to them that you gave a full confession before midnight," I said and fell back to sleep quickly.

The next morning, woken up by the loudspeaker broadcast, I was startled to discover that my roommate was leaning over my bed and staring straight at me. "Are you going to tell them?" she said to me.

"I'll go and tell them right now," I said. I jumped out of bed without delay and hurried off to report to the tiger-hunting group.

"Did she confess before or after the midnight?" Commissar Feng asked me.

"Before midnight. I was very tired last night so I decided to come this morning," I said.

"At what time did she confess?"

"About eleven thirty."

My roommate's husband was immediately expelled from the army and sentenced to several years in jail.

One case had become a standing joke in 201 Division. A cook in the kitchen squad was among one of those accused. He confessed that before the Korean War, he kept a few coins when he shopped in the market for the canteen. The interrogators, unsatisfied with a confession about such a petty crime, pushed the cook to divulge more serious wrongdoing. The interrogation tactic called "rotating wheel" — sleep deprivation — was commonly used. It involved several interrogators taking turns to question one suspect around-the-clock until they exhausted him. After several sleepless days and nights, the cook finally confessed to a more serious crime.

"I confess," he said. "I started the Pacific War." The case was suspended pending further evidence.

The civilians also went through the same political cam-paign. I learned that a local steelworker attempted suicide by thrusting a red-hot iron rod into his stomach after being forced to confess to an embezzlement charge. His intestines were damaged but he healed very quickly because the hot iron bar had been sterilized.

The 200 Division had also rounded up some suspects in the camp. The widow of the division commander, who was killed in the Korean War, was among the suspects. She was a secretary in charge of classified documents. A family "friend" had reported that before going to Korea he had seen the com-mander and his wife counting a "bag of gold" during a visit. In reality, when he walked into the room he actually only saw them putting one gold ring into the bag but he didn't know what else was in it. The commander's widow claimed that it was just a gold ring and a gold-plated watch that she had already handed in to the tiger-hunting group. But they were not convinced and insisted that she surrender the bag of gold. They forced her to kneel down for hours at a time each day on some small rocks in the office. After the prolonged torture, she could hardly stand up or walk. She realized that she would be subjected to the same interrogation day in and day out since there was no such bag of gold to surrender. Already, she was emotionally fragile because her husband had just been killed in the war. There was only one way out of this misery.

One morning she told the babysitter who was taking care of her two daughters to go buy some groceries. When the babysitter returned, she found the commander's wife had committed sui-cide by cutting the big artery in her neck. The blood had spurted out onto the portrait of Chairman Mao on the wall and onto her late husband's picture on the desk. What could have made a loving mother abandon her two young children? Just imagine what kind of constant physical and mental torment she must have been subjected to.

Her two daughters became orphans. The older one was about five years old. The young one was only two years old and belonged to the younger group of kids at the Red Star Kindergarten, which my son later attended.

In the summer, while the Three-Anti's campaign was raging, Wende's brother came to Tangshan to see me. He called me "sister-in-law" as he entered the room where I was having a meeting. It made me feel quite embarrassed in front of so many people. I told him that we hadn't married yet, so it was not proper to address me that way.

The purpose of his trip was to inform me that Wende's mother was dying and wished to see me, the future daughter-in-law once before she died. At the time, Wende was thousands of miles away in Korea. I agreed to go, but Commissar Feng denied me a leave, saying that the workload was too heavy. Even so, I still had to put up with gossip that I hadn't married yet but already wanted to go see my mother-in-law.

I never did get to see my mother-in-law. I insisted on giving Wende's brother some money when he left. My wage was only thirty yuan a month at the time. A month later, I received a letter in red ink from Wende's brother. At first I thought it was good news because it was written in red ink. Then I found out that it was the local custom to write a letter in red whenever old people have passed away.

Later, one of Wende's colleagues told me that Wende had cried as he held his letter in his hand. I had never seen him cry. He didn't ask for a leave to go back to see his mother when she was critically ill, nor did he ask for a leave to attend her funeral. In a letter to the party committee of the 67 Army, dated April 10, 1972, when he was purged during the Cultural Revolution, he wrote about that time in his life:

For the sake of our homeland and the suffering Korean people, I would rather sacrifice my life and my own interests by postponing my marriage; and at the critical moment of the War to Resist America and Aid Korea, I voluntarily gave up the thought of going back to see my mother who fell seriously ill and passed away shortly afterward . . .

Near the end of the Three-Anti's, Commissar Feng summoned me into his office. The air in the office was filled with the mixed smells of smoke and jasmine tea.

"We have had great success in the Three-Anti's campaign. We have uncovered a plot by many officials who had tried to corrupt our party and society. Comrade Qunying, you have done a wonderful job," the commissar said.

"I do what I can, Commissar." I had the feeling that this was not really what he was trying to say.

"How many years have we known each other, Qunying?" His tone of voice suddenly changed.

"We go way back."

"Do you trust me?"

"Of course."

"There's something I want to talk to you about. I have to be honest with you."

Just as I had expected.

Commissar Feng leaned closer, lowering his voice. I could smell the stink of breath mixed with smoke. "You have to prepare yourself for this. Your fiancé, Han Wende, has confessed to embezzling two thousand yuan. He is a big tiger. It is a very serious matter. It is time for you to expose him and draw a clear line with him."

I was in shock and couldn't say anything. That explained why I hadn't received any letter from Wende.

"How could that be possible? He is a very honest person," I said.

"You've only known him a couple of years. There are a lot of things you don't know about him. He has a very complicated history. You should trust our party and organization. We have never wronged an innocent person."

"But I don't know anything about it."

"Well, think carefully. What did he give you when you two met? Did he give you a gold ring?"

"No. He gave me a picture of himself and I gave him a pen. Nothing else."

"That's not what I heard. Can you guarantee you don't know anything?"

"Yes."

"With what?"

"If I'm lying, you can expel me from the army or just shoot me."

"You should trust our party and do a self-examination to think things through. Let me know if you come up with something."

I was temporarily relieved of my job, ordered to write a full confession, and not allowed to leave the camp without permission. I didn't want to believe that Wende was capable of such wrongdoing, but I had started to suspect something was going on. Did the matchmaker eventually succeed in dragging him down? Should I place my complete trust in the party as the commissar had suggested? I wished that I could talk face-to-face with Wende and clear things up. For several months I had been running up and down, collecting information and investigating people; but in the end, I myself became a suspect.

During the eight-month period since I had joined the study group, Wende and I had been completely out of touch with each other, until the day when Wende's old comrade Shouyi returned from the Korean battlefield as a war hero. He was awarded a first-class merit citation and instantly promoted up three ranks. Since he was an illiterate, they sent him to an "instant high school" to study.

When I met Shouyi in the canteen at lunchtime, he bombarded me with questions. "Have you received Wende's letters? He hasn't heard from you since you came back home. He has been very worried. What's going on?"

"I was wondering the same thing. I haven't received any letters from him either. How is he?" I asked.

"He's fine."

Then I revealed all of the details about Wende's embezzlement charge. The comrade's look of surprise quickly changed to amusement.

"No, no," he said. "There's no such thing. Everything's fine. In fact, it's just the opposite. Wende has won a third-class merit citation for diligence and dedication to his work. Don't worry about it." He laughed.

In Korea, because of his dedication to his work and his excellent bookkeeping, Wende had won the merit citation and been promoted to a rank equal to a battalion commander. He didn't tell the party that the matchmaker had tried to convince him to join an embezzling scheme. Betrayal was not one of his qualities. When the embezzling plot was uncovered, only one low-ranking officer was made a scapegoat and the rest went untouched. All my anxiety and suspicion in the past eight months was for nothing, I thought to myself. I felt so guilty that I'd felt a slight doubt about him, but I had known in my heart the whole time that he was a good man. It seemed that they purposely separated couples like us in order to get us to turn on each other; however, I had stood up to the test.

At the end of the Three-Anti's, when they couldn't find anything wrong with Wende and me, they returned all the letters he had sent to me over that period of time. All of the letters had been opened and thoroughly inspected by the officials. There was an enormous bundle. They seemed so heavy to me. I spent the whole night reading them again and again; the handwriting was so familiar and heartwarming. The numerous letters I had written to Wende were also released to him. In fact, he was probably reading them at the same time. Although I was in China and he was in Korea, I felt the distance between us had shortened.

After the Three-Anti's, they didn't send me back to Korea, but instead transferred me to the clinic at the "instant high school" where the war hero Shouyi was studying. He was supposed to write an application for joining the Communist Party after learning how to write, but he never did. He hated to study. Teachers rarely found him in the classroom. He often went outside the campus to watch movies or operas, even though the rules clearly forbade soldiers to do so. But no one dared to confront him because of his war hero status and his bad temper. The officials had to make an exception for him when it came time to write the application. We didn't really need to go out for shopping or entertainment because there was an army shop right on the campus and movies were shown on the weekends. Soviet movies were most common.

In March 1953, Stalin suddenly died. It was said that the crowd attending his funeral in Red Square was so large that many people were crushed to death. Nobody died during the memorial services in China, but there were a lot of people who fainted. All the officials in the camp attended our service, wearing black armbands. We had to stand in a silent tribute with our heads down for one whole hour. Many senior officials, including Commissar Feng, collapsed after observing only thirty minutes of silence. They dropped to the ground, one by one, like trees being chopped down. I was kept busy rescuing them.

A month later, I became a member of the Communist Party. Two comrades had recommended me for membership — a candidate always needed two existing party members to be his or her sponsors when applying for membership. At the induction, I raised my right fist, and, in front of the sickle-and-hammer of the party flag, swore to fight for the just cause of Communism and to be prepared to sacrifice my life for it at any time.

8

THE 38TH PARALLEL AND THE WEDDING

BEGINNING IN THE SUMMER of 1951, the war entered a stalemate stage. The lengthy peace talks started while the war raged on. Even though there was little advancement made by either side, casualties continued to mount. Sometimes the troops would maintain a stronghold at any cost, only to be ordered to give it up the next day.

It was said that in the last two years of the war, the two sides had built the longest, strongest, and most complicated fortification ever. At the frontline, from east to west, tens of thousands of Chinese soldiers built the world's largest underground defense system. The cubic meters of earth and stone they used was said to be enough to build several of the Suez Canal. The shelters were all connected, many built with big logs. They alternated one layer of logs and one layer of soil to a total of six layers of each. A layer was one meter thick, which made the fortifications more than ten meters thick, ensuring that there would be no problem when bombs were dropped. Beds were also constructed of logs with dried grass arranged on top. The higher-ranking officers lived in smaller, more private shelters with fewer people, whereas the common soldiers had to endure large cramped quarters that could each house a whole battalion.

Soon the news came that on the night of July 27, 1953, both sides underwent the heaviest fire of the war. The illuminating shells, signal flares, and artillery fire shook the entire Korean Peninsula. Abruptly, at 10 p.m., the fighting came to a complete standstill. According to some soldiers who came back from Korea, the American soldiers could be seen dancing on the south side of the 38th parallel at a distance that could have been easily covered by handgun fire. The war seemed over. An armistice — a ceasefire agreement had been reached. But it wasn't a peace treaty. Technically, the Korean Peninsula remains in a state of war. The ironic thing was that the war started at the 38th parallel, and, after so many people died on both sides, it ended at the same 38th parallel. The war devastated the entire Korean Peninsula. So many bombs were dropped and rockets expended that some say even today if you randomly reach into the soil, there is a good chance that you will find shrapnel. Casualties on both sides were massive. In three years nearly 37,000 Americans lost their lives according to the U.S. Department of Defense. The Chinese combatant deaths are still a mystery. There are several conflicting claims. The Western sources estimate 900,000. There is an enormous gap comparing that number to the Chinese official sources who reported only 110,000 killed in action, and 35,000 who died from disease. Nevertheless, the Chinese government claimed victory. Even though it is still debatable if the Chinese involvement in the war was necessary at all, one thing that is clear is that this war was the best manifestation of Mao's Human Sea strategy — using overwhelming numbers of people against an enemy who possessed modern weapons. He knew that if he put enough Chinese through the meat grinder, it would eventually jam. He put no value on human lives.

The day after the ceasefire, the troops began withdrawing from the area. With two bodyguards by his side, a regimental commander expressed a desire to stay for another day. "The war is now over; I think it's okay to sleep in the shelter one more night!" That night, the shelter collapsed. One heavy log toppled down, tragically falling on the commander's head. He died instantly.

In early May 1954, I was on the train to Korea for the second time, this time to get married. Almost one year after the war ended, the leaders from the headquarters had finally approved my marriage to Wende.

The 201 Division was one of the troops still stationed in North Korea after the war. It took me a week to get to Wende. Since I had written a letter to him in advance, I knew that he would be expecting me. After a train ride that seemed to last forever, I disembarked wearily at a small railway station. No one had come to meet me. Usually there was a truck from Wende's department that came to the station once a day, but there was no sign of it that day. It was very quiet.

I waited till it got dark. When a truck from the 20th Garrison Division luckily showed up, the men advised me that there wouldn't be any other truck coming along that day. It would therefore be best, they said, if I went with them and they escorted me to Wende's troop later. I had no other choice but to go with them.

That troop was a great distance from Wende's, much farther than I had expected. In fact, we had to travel across several mountains to get to the destination. They were very hospitable, treating me like a guest. After staying for several days, I finally said, "I have to go back to report to my troop." They told me they would arrange a truck to take me there, but it took almost a week for them to do so. On the day of my departure, they had two soldiers accompany me to ensure I made it safely.

Upon my arrival, I found Wende pacing back and forth, his hands placed nervously behind his back. He had worried ceaselessly for several days and had gotten blisters on the corners of his mouth due to anxiety. Even though the war was over, it wasn't safe by any means for a woman to travel alone in a foreign country.

"I thought you got lost or something," he said to me. I had never seen him so worried before. After I finished relating my story, he sighed in relief. After more than two years apart, we were finally reunited.

Wende and I were married that same month. The flowers were everywhere in the springtime, with blossoms appearing first on the trees before the leaves sprung out. After the war, the troops hadn't wasted time moving from the gloomy bomb shelters to the outside where they had built many wooden houses.

"Our young Han is getting married. We've got to prepare a bridal room for the couple," the leader of the supply department said with his Shanxi accent. He immediately ordered twelve soldiers to haul a cabin, constructed of wood, to the south side of the mountain where it would get the most sun. That was very considerate of him. The cabin was sparely decorated with a wooden bed and table, both of which were attached to the floorboards with bolts. The soldiers were also instructed to collect some wildflowers and design some bright wedding decorations.

With the war over, the soldiers were left with nothing to do, so when the news spread about the wedding, all the soldiers decided to attend. The wedding started at six o'clock in the evening and lasted until midnight. The ceremony was held in the meeting hall, which was also built with logs. The hall was illuminated by a gas lamp that was as bright as a hundred-watt lightbulb. Since all the guests had brought wildflowers, the hall was soon alive with color. Most of the soldiers had to stand outside as the celebration started.

Wende was quite awkward in this kind of situation, for he could not easily display affection in public. During the entire wedding, he ignored me completely while he socialized with everyone else, afraid of leaving the guests out in the cold. I felt like I was marrying a stranger.

At the time, there were three sizes of "kitchens" available — the large size was for the masses of common soldiers, the medium size was for the slightly more important officers, and the small private kitchens were reserved for high officials. That festive night, Wende and I enjoyed the "small kitchen." The main dish was tofu, a secret recipe the cook had invented. It tasted very sour because of the wild grapes that were used as ferment. After leaving Korea, I was never able to eat tofu for the rest of my life. The wedding banquet also included some bitter wild vegetables sprinkled with salt, plenty of candy, and some strong liquor from China. It didn't take long for the officials to get Wende drunk, since he couldn't handle much alcohol. He hadn't drunk or smoked in his whole life.

"Now we have finally defeated the American imperialists and Korea is at peace . . ." Commissar Feng gave a speech that made me feel like I was at a political meeting rather than my own wedding. "Wende is a good comrade, diligent and honest. We all know that he has done a wonderful job during the Three-Anti's movement and won a third-class merit citation . . ."

Then he suggested that we tell our love story. "It's the tradition for the newlyweds to tell their love story. From the very beginning. Comrade Wende, you start first," he said.

"Yes, don't leave any details out," someone yelled.

"There's nothing to tell," Wende said. His face was all red from the liquor.

"Comrade Qunying, you tell us," the commissar said.

"I don't have anything to tell either," I said.

"Come on. Give us something, anything," someone in the crowd said.

"Well, I . . ." I stuttered. For a moment I felt like I was under interrogation. "Do you want to hear the true story? Alright, we handed in our marriage application four years ago and permission was not granted. Why?"

Commissar Feng and the rest of the officials sat in stony silence, their faces grim.

"That's the past already. Let's not talk about it," Wende interrupted me. "Yes. Let's talk about something else," someone echoed, trying to restore the lighthearted mood.

Wende had never complained in his whole life. "The party and organization had their reasons," he said.

PART II

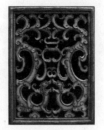

9

Peace

AFTER THE WAR, the officers at regimental level were allowed to bring their wives into Korea to live with them. I was ordered to go to the border to meet the wives and bring them army uniforms to wear because civilians were not allowed to enter the country. Some of the wives were rather young while others appeared to be getting on in years. The wife of the commander of the Third Regiment was an old woman with small bound feet. It looked quite strange to see her small triangle-shaped feet poking out from beneath the baggy uniform. I had to put a pair of army boots over her tiny shoes so they wouldn't cause suspicion at the border. I went back and forth twice and brought forty wives over.

It was about that time when I started feeling sick for some unknown reason. In August, a high-ranking officer had become ill and had to go back to China for a checkup. A nurse and I were assigned to accompany him. I thought it would be a good opportunity to have a health check as well.

After my arrival in Beijing, I promptly went to see a doctor. To my surprise, he informed me that I was not sick, but pregnant. We stayed in an army guest house in *Nanchizi*, on the east side of the Imperial Palace where emperors once resided and ruled. During my twenty-day stay in Beijing, I had a chance to eat all the things I craved, which I could never get a hold of in Korea. That was the advantage of eating in the· canteen for high-ranking officials. The officer, the nurse, and I had one table to ourselves and enjoyed four dishes with rice every meal. Sometimes we had steamed meat-stuffed buns. I often went out to browse through stores along the street. The sight of clothes and cosmetics was very tempting. Of course, we were forbidden to use any of these products, not even face cream or soap with fragrance, which was considered a part of bourgeoisie lifestyle. My wage was very low at the time so I didn't have enough money to buy such things anyway. Nevertheless, I proudly walked down the street in army uniform and drew a lot of respect and attention. While wandering around, I noticed a poster for the Beijing opera's performance of *Geifei Zuijiu* — Geifei Intoxicated, starring Mei Lanfang. I returned to the guest house and casually mentioned to the officer over supper that I was a big fan of Beijing opera from a very young age, but the tickets were so expensive that I could never afford them. The officer volunteered to buy tickets for the nurse and me. At first we didn't want to accept the expensive gift, but he insisted.

Because I had heard of Mei Lanfang since I was young it was exciting to see him in person in the grand theater, with dazzling lights and a crimson velvet curtain. There were many high-ranking army officers and rich people in the audience. Average people couldn't afford such a luxury. The play was frequently accompanied by cheers and applause. Mei Lanfang played Geifei — a highest-ranking imperial concubine. I couldn't tell that Mei was a man by his appearance and voice.

Mei Lanfang was one of the most famous Beijing opera performers, well known for his *qingyi* — female roles. He was the first artist to introduce Beijing opera to foreign countries. During the eight-year Anti-Japanese War, he withdrew from the stage, refused to perform for the Japanese troops, and grew a beard to ruin his feminine image. He passed away before the Cultural Revolution during which many artists were persecuted.

After having a wonderful time in Beijing, I returned to Korea. When Wende heard the good news that I was pregnant, he was very happy and told me to take good care of myself. As my pregnancy went on, he started to worry. Since we lived halfway up the mountain and I often went out to lend a hand at the clinic located at the foot of the mountain, he was afraid that I might slip and fall on the steep paths. Spies in the area gave him another reason to worry. Because there was not much for him to do after the war, he often followed me around wherever I went.

After the war, the food got better and it wasn't dropped from planes, but was shipped by trucks. The principal food was canned fish and cured meat. There were still no fresh vegetables. So I often collected edible wild vegetables to eat.

During the three years of war, all the Korean cities and villages had been bombed to the ground. Most Korean families were left without men, since so many of them were in the army or had been killed in battle. Chinese troops assisted the Koreans to rebuild and had frequent contact with the locals. Since Korea was a Japanese colony for many years, the Koreans could speak some Japanese. With the few Japanese words I had learned in school, I could carry on some basic conversation with them. "You Japanese slave," an old Korean woman said to me jokingly and laughed.

At the beginning of 1955, when I was nine months' pregnant, the 201 Division had already started withdrawing from Korea; however, the doctors thought that I would be wise to wait until the baby was born. I waited for many days, but nothing happened. By February, when I still hadn't given birth, I decided to leave, thinking that there would be a hospital in Pyongyang or Andong. The trip went without incident, even with all the jostling I went through in the truck as we drove along the bumpy mountain roads. Wende worried all the way home.

When we crossed the Yalu River and arrived back in the homeland in Andong, we transferred onto a civilian train to Jinan, the capital city of Shangdong Province. From there we changed trains to Jiaoxian County, and from there we went to

Jiaonan County by truck. The majority of the troop came back in a cargo train with vents only on the roofs. No one knew where they were going until they arrived in Jinan to have lunch.

Upon our arrival back in China, the 201 Division was stationed in Jiaonan County. Soldiers were welcomed at home as heroes returned from the battlefield and were respectfully called "the dearest people." Officials in the local government invited the heroes to watch opera. There was no military camp at the time and the troop had to board with the locals while the camp was under construction. There I stayed for about two months without giving birth.

When labor finally commenced, it kept me in the local hospital for four days with severe pain. Since I was undergoing a difficult labor at the age of thirty-one, which was considered risky, the local doctors were afraid that they couldn't handle the situation and suggested that I should be transferred to the Second Hospital of 67 Army in Jiaoxian County. I was quickly taken by military truck to the Second Hospital, fifty miles away.

The next day when the baby still refused to make an appearance, the army doctor decided to perform a Caesarean section, to which I reluctantly agreed. The doctors had Wende sign an agreement to state that if they could save only one, save the adult. He was more anxious than I was, but there was nothing he could do to help. At the last possible moment, when I was already lying on the operating table, my abdomen sterilized with alcohol, I changed my mind and jumped off the table.

"There has to be a better way," I said.

I refused to have the procedure. They got a hold of a specialist who assured me that I would be fine and advised me to wait a few more days. In the meantime, they would monitor my condition closely.

The baby was already two months overdue, so what difference would another day or two make, I thought to myself. By that time, I hadn't slept for six days due to the agonizing pain, so they gave me some kind of sedative to help me rest. In the afternoon, I experienced piercing contractions. At ten o'clock that night, my baby finally decided to come into this world after eleven months and eight days in his mother's womb. The doctor held the baby close to my face. "Look, you got a fat son."

I lay in the ward feeling very weak but peaceful during those spring days. We named the baby Xianping, meaning "Korea at peace." Entering the hospital room, Wende felt quite happy yet a little sentimental.

"When will this little thing grow up?" he said.

While the new military camp was under construction, we stayed with a local family. The couple had had an opium business before liberation. After discovering that she couldn't give birth, the woman bought a girl so that when she grew up she could take care of the business. After liberation, the opium trade became illegal so the couple closed their business. The old woman was very abusive toward the girl, who was fifteen at the time, so the girl often came over to talk about it with me. "I want to get out of here and go with you," she said to me. "I can do anything for you."

"I'm just looking for a babysitter for my son; I'll go back to work very soon. Would you like to take care of him for me? I'll pay you a good wage, higher than any other babysitter," I said. I really needed a babysitter at the time.

"Sure, I'd like to," she said.

"See if your mother agrees," I said.

"It's none of her business. She's not my mother. They bought me and wanted me to serve those opium users," she said.

"Where are your real parents?"

"They live very nearby here. They sold me, so I don't care about them. I want to go with you."

When the stepmother heard the news, she was very upset. "You ungrateful little bitch! You'd have starved to death without me. Go and serve your goddamn Communist master! Don't ever come back here again," she yelled. The old lady hated Communists, never missing an opportunity to say so.

A few months later, the construction of the military camp was complete. The camp was surrounded by high walls with broken glass along the top to prevent people from climbing over. The poor children from a nearby village often came scrounging for garbage. With nothing to do during the day the war hero Shouyi often walked around the camp chasing the "wild kids" away.

Shortly after we moved into the new camp, some army horses suddenly died for an unknown reason. They were buried outside the wall. When the destitute villagers nearby got wind of it, they dug the carcasses up and divided the horse meat among themselves. The entire village was poisoned and sent to the hospital.

In June, three months after Xianping was born, the order came to demobilize female soldiers. Many of them had already taken off their uniforms and gone home to become housewives. No matter how hard they tried to persuade me to become a housewife, I firmly refused. I was not cut out for that. I told them that I couldn't handle it. I had joined the army when I was eighteen — before I had ever mastered the skills of housework.

In July, I was forced to say goodbye to my army life, but I still refused to become a housewife. Instead I asked to be transferred to Jiaonan County Hospital where I finally became a real doctor. The hospital was divided into the departments of Internal Medicine (physician), Surgery (surgeon), Gynecology and Obstetrics, Pediatrics, X-rays, Dentistry, Ophthalmology, ENT (ear, nose, throat), and so on. Out of the one hundred or so doctors in the hospital, there were only thirty who had university educations. The rest just had basic medical training. The old doctor in the Traditional Chinese Medicine Department had never had any formal education. His skills were handed down in his family for generations. I was one of the two doctors who was transferred from the army. I had only had training here and there. And mostly my experience was of amputating arms and legs on the battlefield. I had to work and study at the same time. Hospitals below the county level usually didn't possess any doctors with university education at all. That was the reality in China. I was assigned to work as a physician in the Internal Medicine Department — the first stop for outpatients who would be referred to other departments if necessary. The hospital was about ten miles away from Wende's army camp. I had my own room in the hospital dorm and only visited Wende on the weekend or during my day off after the night shift. Sometimes Wende would come to the hospital to visit me and the baby. It was a nice coastal town in Shangdong Peninsula, never getting overly hot in the summer.

Shortly after I said goodbye to my army life, Wende came home one day, wearing a brand new Soviet-style uniform, formally ranked lieutenant. Under the Soviet influence, the army changed its uniforms to Soviet style, and the military ranks were standardized. In the 1950s, the Soviet Union was China's closest ally though the relationship was marked by distrust from the very beginning. Mao and Stalin had differences dating back to the 1930s over Mao's guerrilla war strategy. Nevertheless, the Soviets — "big brother" — sent thousands of technical advisers to help industrialize and modernize China. Many Chinese students were sent to the Soviet Union to study. Russian music and songs became very popular in China at the time. The new uniform made Wende look dignified. He had three stars on his epaulets.

"We are no longer the rustic Eighth Route Army — no more ragged uniforms," he said proudly.

"Too bad I never got the chance to wear the new one," I said.

Wende went straight to the baby, picked him up, and marched around and around the house. The baby fell asleep in his arms within two minutes.

"It's funny that every time I come home to see the baby, he's sleeping," he said.

"Well, stop pacing around. You make him sleepy. Talk to him," I said. But Wende didn't know any baby talk.

After I started working in the hospital, the girl came to babysit Xianping. Her stepmother came to visit sometimes, and I treated her with respect, and served her with tea and cigarettes. Since the famous Longjing tea was difficult to come by, Wende and I always saved it for our guests. "I can't taste the difference between the famous tea and the average," Wende often said to me. Even though we never smoked, we always kept a supply of cigarettes on hand for company. It was a social standard to offer guests cigarettes — it didn't matter if the guest smoked or not, it would be considered to be inhospitable, perhaps even an insult, if you didn't make the offer. Because some guests refused the offer just to be *keqi* — a Chinese way of being polite — you had to offer many times while repeatedly saying, "Make yourself at home" even after the guests said no many times. This tradition is still in place today.

When the fragrance of Longjing tea and the pungent smell of smoke began to circulate through the air, the old woman would start her long tirade of curses. "You know, Qunying, if it were not for the goddamn Commies, I would still have my business. In fact, I would still be rich. It was a very lucrative business. Those sons of bitches ruined it for me," she said. She took a deep puff, breathed out the smoke, and took a sip of tea. "Say, this is good tea." She had a discriminating taste when it came to tea.

At first I tried to ignore her grumbles, thinking she was just an ignorant old woman, not even bothering to argue with her. I thought our Communist army had saved the people from a miserable life in the evil old society. And here I entertained her with fine tea and cigarettes while she was condemning the Communists. I could only stand so much before I decided to comment on the old lady's rude behavior.

"I am a Communist, you know," I finally said to her.

"I know that, but you are a good Commie. You are different from them," the old woman said in a matter-of-fact tone. "But those sons of . . . ." She never stopped swearing at the Communists.

The young babysitter was a hard worker. She took care of Xianping, and at the same time cooked and washed clothes. I gave her the highest wage among the babysitters in the neighborhood. Since she ate with us, she could save all of her earnings. All of the other babysitters were very jealous of her because they made much less and had to eat separately from their "masters." The "masters" only gave their babysitters leftovers to eat. How could they take advantage of those poor country girls?

When Xianping was about four months old, sixty local peasants got food poisoning from seafood and I worked non-stop throughout the night rescuing all of them. My son didn't get fed and cried all night. The young babysitter carried him around the house, crying as well, not knowing what to do.

Wende had received a letter from his brother Guangde, who wanted to leave the countryside to find a job here with us in the hospital. In the early fifties, it was easier to find a job and transfer *hukou* — residence registration. Near the end of July, Guangde arrived along with his wife and their son, who was about Xianping's age. Guangde took a job as an accountant in the hospital. The two brothers both had patience with numbers. Guangde's wage was twenty-four yuan a month, which was the standard average worker's salary. Considering that he had just started, it wasn't all that bad. At the time, I was paid sixty-three yuan a month after many years of revolution. Guangde's wife was a housewife. She stayed home and cooked. We lived together peacefully for some time.

Guangde's wife was the type of country woman who would get homesick in three days if she didn't see the smoke coming out of the chimney of her own house. Soon we started to have occasional brushes over one trivial thing or another. She made some unreasonable demands. She wanted me to hire a babysitter for her son too. But I told her that our babysitter could take care of both of the babies when she was cooking. We had a carriage that could fit two babies. Then she didn't want the babysitter to eat with us and told Guangde: "I didn't come here to cook for the babysitter. And you are only earning a babysitter's wage. We still have to depend on your brother." So I had no choice but to let the girl eat at the canteen to avoid the problem. I gave the babysitter fifteen yuan a month while she was eating with us, so she could save all her wages. When she started eat at the canteen, I increased her wage. One day I gave the girl some dumplings to eat and it made Guangde's wife very upset.

During that time, Guangde contracted malaria transmitted by mosquitoes. His symptoms included shivering and a high fever every day, sometimes every other day. Afraid of passing it on to the children, I had to put him in quarantine by finding another place for him to stay. "You see, when you are sick, they kick you out!" Guangde's wife said to him. It took more than twenty days for Guangde to overcome his illness. A few months later, when the Chinese New Year was approaching, Guangde had a talk with me. His wife insisted on going back to their hometown for the festival and she didn't plan to come back. He was facing a dilemma. "What should I do, sister?" he asked me. He talked in a slow and mild tone just like his brother Wende did.

"We have arranged everything for you. We can't decide this for you. You have to make up you own mind," I said to him.

Guangde's family only stayed for about six months before they returned home for the New Year and never came back. Wende gave me many lectures on how to get along with relatives during that time. The conflict between Guangde's wife and me didn't end there, but was to be continued ten years later when we would come face to face again.

Every time I worked the nightshift, I would get the next day off. Sometimes my day off coincided with Sunday so I would take the baby and the young babysitter to see Wende at his army camp ten miles away. A copy clerk in Wende's 601 Regiment, liked the babysitter and sent a matchmaker to talk to me. At first, they didn't know the girl was a babysitter because I treated her just like a member of my family. After the girl was introduced to the soldier, she immediately agreed to the marriage. The clerk was young and not bad looking. I felt happy for her, but the marriage left me without someone to look after my baby.

I had to find another babysitter at once. The new girl was nineteen. When I took her and the baby to see Wende, a warehouseman in the army camp fell in love with the girl and sent a matchmaker to talk to me. Even though the warehouseman was an honest and dependable man, he was already forty years old and had big black pockmarks all over his face. Their marriage left me without a babysitter once again.

It was very difficult for me to handle my busy work schedule without a babysitter. Wende wrote to his family in his hometown for help. His second sister, who had health problems, said to his third sister: "If I didn't have a disease, I would go to take care of the boy. That's our brother's first child." In the beginning of 1956, Wende's third sister came all the way from Heibei Province to care for Xianping. She was just like Wende, very gentle and a slow talker. She was very diligent, babysitting, cooking, and even making baby shoes for Xianping, a craft that many country women possessed. The baby shoes always fit perfectly and over time they were getting bigger and bigger. She even made shoes for me. Those handmade shoes felt very comfortable. They were carefully sewn by hand, thread by thread. She only stayed for a few months and then returned home.

After Wende's sister left, I found a fifty-one-year-old babysitter from the countryside. I decided that older women were more dependable than young girls. I called her "Sister Liu," a polite form of address for an older woman. She looked much older than her age. I could tell that she'd had a very hard life. She was of medium height with a long, thin face that looked quite kind. She had a pair of small bound feet and her pockmarked face revealed that she had been a survivor of smallpox. Smallpox was a highly contagious and often fatal disease that causes a skin rash and scabs. For centuries, epidemics of smallpox killed millions of people worldwide and was once regarded as a major health threat, but was eradicated by the end of the seventies through immunization. The World Health Organization declared the eradication of the disease in 1980. It became the first communicable disease to ever have been eradicated. And now people don't know much about it anymore.

"I got married at the age of seventeen, gave birth to a son at eighteen, and became a young widow at nineteen," Sister Liu said. "I have never married again since then — it's the tradition. My mother-in-law promised to set up my *zhen jie pai* for remaining chaste to my dead husband. My late husband had a restaurant while he was alive. After he died, the restaurant closed and we became very poor. Now I'm working as a babysitter. You are the fourth family I've worked for. Don't be fooled by my age: I'm very strong, I can do a lot of work."

The first day she came, she didn't want to eat with us. "When I worked for the other families, I always ate separately from them. I just eat whatever is left," the old nanny said.

"Come eat with us. I don't care how they treated you before — here you'll have to eat with us," I said to her.

"It's the custom for women to eat leftovers after everyone else is done with their meal. Men and women shouldn't even sit together at the same table," the old nanny said.

"In our new society, men and women are equal now," I said to her.

The old babysitter finally sat at the table after repeated invitations. When Xianping was about three years old, he discovered a secret about the old babysitter. "Mom, why does Auntie have only one toe?" he whispered to me while he was lying in the bed one night.

"One toe?"

"Yes, I saw it when she was washing her feet."

Since the old babysitter had a pair of bound feet, she always washed her deformed feet in private to avoid being seen by people, but Xianping discovered this secret by chance. Because the four small toes were pressed down in the direction of the sole of the foot during the foot-binding procedure, it appeared as though there was only one big toe on her foot. The matter was too complex, and loaded with too much history, to explain to a young child. He wouldn't understand.

Xianping also had nightmares during that time because the old nanny always told scary stories about tigers and ghosts. "Sister Liu," I said to the babysitter, "Xianping is growing older, and will understand these stories and easily get frightened, so don't tell such stories anymore."

"Okay, I won't anymore. I've run out of stories anyway. That's all I've got," the babysitter replied. She did not speak of superstitions again for a while, but when she did it would be at a crucial moment.

10

Tiger's Teeth

In the spring of 1956, Chairman Mao issued his newest proposal of "Let a hundred flowers bloom, let a hundred schools of
thought contend" to permit greater intellectual and artistic
freedom as an effort to encourage the participation of the intellectuals in the new society. "The spring is here, let a hundred
flowers bloom," Chairman Mao proposed at a Supreme State
Conference on May 2, 1956. "Within the limit of the
Constitution of the People's Republic of China, everyone
should be allowed to express their thoughts freely without any
interference. Two thousand years ago during the Spring and
Autumn Period, everyone was allowed to express their opinions
freely and saw a proliferation of new ideas and philosophies.
That's what we need now."

Those were busy days. We had to get up at four or five
o'clock in the morning, then head straight to the office for
drawn-out political meetings where we listened to someone
read newspapers until six o'clock. Afterward, we would return
home to have breakfast and leave for work at seven. At night,
the political meeting would last till eleven or twelve. The hospital leaders didn't seem to care if people dozed off during the
long meetings as long as everyone showed up.

At the hospital meeting, President Ding strongly encouraged
people to speak freely as the movement intended, but instead he
was faced with complete silence. Everyone was acting just like

elementary school students, who couldn't come up with any answers and thought that disaster had fallen upon them. However, with the repeated invitation from the leaders, people started to open up. In the end, there was an outburst of complaints and criticism directed toward the Communist Party and society. It turned out that a majority of the people had something to grumble about. It looked like no one was satisfied with the new society that we had sacrificed and fought for. Wende was very worried after I told him about the meeting.

"I hope you didn't say anything outrageous," he said, knowing me as one who liked to speak out without thinking carefully.

"Everyone had to take turns to say something. I had no choice. I made some suggestions," I said. "After all, when does the average person have a chance to say anything? I said that bureaucracy still existed in our hospital today. We are the people's hospital and are supposed to serve the people, yet some doctors still treat patients, especially those from the countryside, very rudely. Some leaders in our hospital only care about themselves and get things done by using their pull. We should put an end to this kind of behavior."

"Think twice before you say anything," he said.

"I never thought about it before, but the ones complaining might be right," I said. "Dr. Chen said that not everything Chairman Mao says is right. No one can be right all the time. Even the sun is not completely red, there's a black spot on it."

Dr. Chen had a university education and seemed to know a lot. Another doctor complained that there were too many political meetings and if doctors didn't try to improve their professional ability, how could they serve the people? Some people complained that the wages were too low.

In June of 1957, when I was several months' pregnant with my second baby, Bingbing, the Hundred Flowers movement came to an abrupt halt after the government issued a mandate to "muster our force to defeat rightists' frenzied attacks." It signaled the start of the Anti-Rightist movement, a major witch hunt against intellectuals. The hospital immediately formed an investigation group to hunt down the rightists. Anyone who had spoken out during the Hundred Flowers movement would now be considered a rightist.

President Ding asked how people could have done such a contemptible thing when the Communist Party had liberated them from the evils of the old society. Instead of expressing gratitude, they had viciously attacked the party. This was described as "eating when you pick up the bowl, but cursing your mother the minute you put it down."

The investigation group uncovered plenty of rightists in the hospital during that time. Dr. Chen's remark that there was a black spot in the sun was held against him. As people "remembered" later, he had said that the sun was black, and he was therefore labeled a rightist. The sun was a symbol of our great leader Chairman Mao. Dr. Chen was banished to the country-side. His wife changed their children's surname to her family name and told the children to call him uncle instead of father so the children could avoid persecution. In Chinese history, people could be punished for being even remotely related to one who had committed a crime. In ancient times, a punishment was commonly called "extermination of the nine degrees of kindred" — the nine generations from one's great-great-grandfather down to one's great-great-grandson. Or some say it means four generations of one's paternal relations, three generations of one's maternal relations, and two generations of one's wife's relations. The purpose was to eliminate anyone who could take revenge, and also to make it the family's and relatives' responsibility to watch each other so that no one committed a crime.

The other young doctor who had complained that there were too many political meetings was marked as a rightist for twenty-two years, during which time no one dared marry him; he was almost fifty years old when he finally married.

People didn't forget the comments I had made either, but I said I hadn't meant anything derogatory by them. I didn't

qualify as a rightist, perhaps because my lack of higher education prevented me from being considered an intellectual.
Nonetheless, it still gave me many sleepless nights.

"I told you," Wende said in a tone mixed with sarcasm and
accusation. In a way, he seemed to be glad that it had happened just so that he could prove he was right, and I hated
when he was right. One might have said something casually,
forgetting about it afterwards; however, people remembered for
you, refreshing your memory when the right time came. They
had good memories.

During the Anti-Rightist movement, every work unit had to
find rightists according to quotas allocated by the higher
authorities. Not being able to fill the quotas was an indication
of failure, whereas surpassing the quotas was considered a tri-
umph. More than a half million of the brightest intellectuals
were publicly humiliated, imprisoned, and banished to the
countryside. The campaign had a huge impact on the party's
policy and later political campaigns. In October 1957, with the
Anti-Rightist campaign escalating, Chairman Mao pointed out
during the third session of the Eighth Party Congress that the
main conflict was still between the proletarian and the bourgeoisie, socialism and capitalism. This was a fundamental
change from the statement a year earlier during the first session of the Eighth Party Congress that "the phase of the class
struggle in a large scale has been completed and the major
work onward will be national reconstruction." In the following
years, Mao called on the party members: "Never forget class
struggle." So the class struggle became the guiding principle for
the party's policy and people's everyday lives. This Anti-Rightist
campaign had paved the way for the Great Leap Forward, the
Four-Cleanups movement, and the Great Cultural Revolution.

Some historians speculated that Mao's proposal of "let a
hundred flowers bloom" was just a trap to get the intellectuals
to open up and then to persecute them. This tactic was a dupli-
cate of one of the *Thirty-Six War Strategies* by the ancient war

strategist Sunzi: "Allow him more latitude first to keep a tighter rein on him afterward." This speculation is logical because Mao was a brilliant war strategist. Others think that after the economic successes of the first years of Communist rule, Mao was overconfident, and believed that he could loosen up the tight reins a bit on free speech. But as soon as the criticism of the party poured in, his tolerance reached its limit. Whatever his original intention was, it certainly didn't end up well.

In December 1957, I gave birth to my second baby, Bingbing. He was born in the army hospital at eight o'clock in the evening. A doctor from another hospital in the 201 Division came to assist with the birth. It went smoothly. After the baby turned one month old, I went back to work.

Early in 1958, when Bingbing was about three or four months old, we all went to a photo studio to have a picture taken. It was wintertime and everyone was bundled up in winter coats, except Bingbing who was wrapped in a quilt. Wende was wearing an impressive army uniform while I wore civilian clothes. My three-year-old son, Xianping, held a pigeon tightly in his small hands. He raised pigeons and rabbits as pets.

Only a few months after this photo was taken, our family was split into three parts. And this wouldn't be the last time we were separated.

In mid 1958, less than a year after the Anti-Rightist movement came the Great Leap Forward movement. Apparently people were doing things too slowly. Following liberation and the Korean War, the nation was still poor, with limited steel production. Mao wanted to leap forward in order to catch up with the advanced steel output of Great Britain in the brief period of a few years — shortened from the originally planned fifteen years. In May 1958, Chairman Mao gave the instruction: "Going all out, aiming high and achieving greater, faster, better, and more economic results to build socialism." Even though the party leaders were generally satisfied with the achievement of the First Five-Year Plan, Mao believed that more could be accomplished in the Second Five-Year Plan with a single step — a great leap forward. It was a frantic and unprecedented mobilization of the peasantry, and mass organizations aimed at achieving economic and technical development at a lightning pace with greater results. Mao used the "human sea strategy" well in the Civil War and Korean War. Then he just applied this same tactic toward economic advancement.

The People's Commune was formed in the countryside to support the Leap. The political meetings in our hospital in those days were all about the three banners: the General Line, the Great Leap Forward, and the People's Commune. Communes were collective units which were divided in turn into production brigades and teams. Private property such as furniture, cooking utensils, animals, and grain were all handed in to the communes for everyone to share. Private cooking was replaced by commune dining, later known as "eating from the same huge pot" — getting the same benefit as everyone else regardless of one's performance in work. This had destroyed the peasants' incentive to work hard. By the end of the year, over 25,000 communes were born across the country, each with an average of 5,000 households.

The small rudimentary steel-making furnaces that were built in the backyard of the communes, became the symbol of the movement. By the end of 1958, there were 600,000 of them built for the purpose of creating steel. People used any type of fuel they could find to power the furnaces, from coal to coffins. Many trees were chopped down to fuel the furnaces, causing enormous environmental damage. There were no environmental protection measures under Mao. The communes melted any iron objects such as pots, pans, bicycles, farming equipment, even door hinges to make steel girders, but these girders were unusable as they were of a low quality. Since all the peasants were eating at the public canteen in those days, there was no need for individuals to have cooking utensils anymore.

Workers, students, and doctors within the town participated in the steelmaking at the five furnaces that were set up a mile north of the hospital. Leaders in the hospital would send about ten people each day to take part in the campaign. They would go around the residential compound to collect metal objects. I had to hand in Bingbing's baby carriage — the frame and wheel were metal. It was also during this time that millions of cadres were sent down to the countryside to do manual labor.

This was also the year a campaign had been launched to exterminate the "four evils": birds, rats, insects, and flies. People in the whole country were organized to create noises, banging drums and pans to prevent sparrows from landing anywhere, until they fell from the sky with exhaustion. In the city, everyone stopped working to gather in the streets, making a racket the whole day through. In the countryside, peasants set up scarecrows in the field while old men, women, and children were made to sit on the edge of the field, zealously beating washbasins. Later on, they said that the birds might be more good than evil since they ate insects too. Without them, the insect population grew rapidly, so people were ordered to stop their massacre. It was another example of wasted effort and mismanagement.

In the countryside, innovative farming and experiments in hybridism were also being conducted. Peasants were engaged in deep plowing and close planting, which leaders believed would enhance crop production. In some cases, they dug more than ten feet deep into the field.

Even the hospital had an experimental field on the east side. Doctors and nurses dug one meter deep into the soil and planted the wheat seeds very closely together. When the next spring rolled around, the wheat stalks grew densely but each was very weak because they were all competing for the limited nutrients in the soil. The nutrients on the surface were buried deep at the bottom during the deep plowing process. As wind swept across the field, the brittle wheat fell to the ground.

It was such a busy time. Going out early in the morning while my children were sleeping, I returned late at night only to find they had already gone to bed. All the doctors and nurses were instructed to work at the furnaces set up nearby, leaving only a few staff on duty at the hospital. The hospital leaders encouraged doctors and nurses to write pledge letters to state that they were willing to give up their weekends and holidays to participate in "voluntary labor."

In summer 1958, because we were preparing for war with Taiwan, all the children in the 67 Army were required to be sent to the Red Star Kindergarten in Qingdao City, on the coast about fifty miles away from home in the Shangdong Peninsula. During that time, China declared its intention to liberate Taiwan, and restarted an extensive artillery shelling of the Nationalist-held islands of Jinmen and Mazu off the coast of Fujian Province in the southeast. The kindergarten was near a beach where people swam in summer. In total, there were about eighty kids of different ages. All the child-care workers were soldiers. Together, Wende and I set out for Qingdao to drop off our son. The weather was quite warm and we bought Xianping a pair of sandals and a T-shirt. Xianping wept quietly and wiped tears away with his hand when we left.

A week after we sent Xianping to the kindergarten, Wende's 201 Division dispatched one battalion to help build a bridge in Jiangsu Province. He would be working there for six months or so. A photo of him with the bridge in the background was taken when the work was completed. This showed the army's involvement in the Great Leap Forward movement.

Almost immediately after Wende left, I was sent by the hospital to the city of Weifang, a hundred miles away, to attend a "class on the continued studies on pulmonary tuberculosis (TB) treatment and prevention." Before that I was sent to Jiaoxian County Hospital to study pediatrics because the doctor from the

Pediatric Department had been transferred somewhere else and they wanted me to replace her. Shortly afterward, the officials changed their minds and sent me to this TB treatment and prevention class at Weifang No. 1 People's Hospital. The trainees were chosen from each county hospital within the province. There was a TB epidemic at the time and I would discover two or three cases each day in the hospital. TB is a chronic bacterial infection that causes more deaths worldwide than any other infectious disease. It has a long history. In the past, it was also called "white plague" because its sufferers appear notably pale. Even during the fifties after some effective antibiotics were invented, it was still considered a fatal disease.

TB is transmitted though coughing, sneezing, or speaking. The disease is characterized by the development of granular tumors, primarily in the lungs. The symptoms include a bloody cough and fever. A chest X-ray was the standard form of diagnosis. Before antibiotics were available, we used traditional Chinese medicine to treat the disease. But from my own experience, I had never seen one TB patient cured by it. At the time, the antibiotic medicine called streptomycin — the first remedy for TB — was most commonly used. It was very expensive — more than two yuan for a small bottle that contained one gram of the medicine. It was in powder form and had to be diluted with distilled water before using — one bottle a day — half in the morning and half in the afternoon. The treatment usually lasted about a week. Long-term use may cause deafness and damage to the nervous system. So the cost of the treatment worked out to be more than fifteen yuan while the standard worker's wage at the time was twenty-four yuan a month. The doctor's wage was about thirty-eight yuan when first practicing. However, the price wasn't the only problem. Because the drug was in extremely short supply and carefully rationed, doctors were only given seven coupons per month to treat their patients. Each coupon was good for just one bottle, which meant that one doctor would only have enough of this drug to treat one TB patient every month. Since I took the advanced training class in Weifang to treat the disease, I was given twice the number of coupons per month.

The other commonly used drug was isoniazid, an oral pill, usually used for about three months. To prevent TB, BCG vaccine was introduced during the fifties and more widely used in post-sixties in China. During that time, Wende's second sister was suffering from TB. I mailed her streptomycin and isoniazid on several occasions, and when I ran out of my streptomycin coupons, I asked other doctors to chip in some of their coupons. That was all I could do for her.

I took Bingbing and the old babysitter with me to Weifang. The three of us lived in a one-room dorm. The old babysitter took care of Bingbing, and in her spare time, she sewed little clothes for the baby by hand. She was good at needlework. She always made her own clothes. She never bought new clothes her whole life. I was supposed to study for a year but because of the lack of staff in the hospital at home, I was called back after about five months. We left around late October when the temperature was cooling off and Bingbing was wearing a sweater.

We studied during the day and participated in steelmaking at night. On an early fall night in 1958, the trainees and the hospital staff including the cooks were sent down to the suburbs to make steel. At a close distance I observed as the trainees unearthed a decades-old grave that some said had good feng shui — in folk belief, the location of a house or tomb has a great influence on the fortune of a family.

"Why are you digging up the grave?" I asked one of my fellow trainees.

"We ran out wood to burn. The coffin can be burned to fuel the furnace," he said.

I never participated in this frenzied event partly because I was raised as a superstitious person even though I never admitted it. According to the elders, digging up ancestral tombs would disturb the feng shui and spirits. Besides, to me it was an immoral thing to do. However, on the other hand, they didn't have a choice — they had run out of things to burn and a quota to meet. So doctors and nurses around my age or older just stood and watched while the very young all participated with great enthusiasm. The peasants — who believed that unearthing graves was the most serious insult toward their ancestors — didn't dare to interfere and just observed nearby. The villagers had built a huge furnace in the field. They gave up farming, and concentrated on steel production. They melted all their farming tools, like ploughshares and picks, even taking off door hinges to assist in the campaign.

The white roots of the shrubs embraced the coffin tightly so they used a shovel to cut through them and pry open the coffin. It sounded as if an old heavy door were being opened. The wooden box had been sealed with big nails.

"Why did they use such big nails on the coffin? Were they afraid that the dead could escape or something?" some joked in the dark.

Ghoulish laughter echoed through the gloomy night.

A young tomb raider swung a lamp closer to the casket. Everyone was astounded at what they saw when the heavy lid was pulled off. A woman lay inside, wearing a bright blue silk skirt and dainty flower-embroidered shoes. I could see everything so vividly. Seconds later, a gust of wind came up, whipping the lady and her dress into dust. When the young people took the coffin apart and threw it into the furnace, it began to make crackling noises that sounded like curses. A putrid odor stung our nostrils. People's faces flickered in the eerie fire. An old peasant was smoking his pipe nearby and stared at the flame listlessly.

At the beginning of 1959, my son Xianping, then five years old, came down with the measles, and I had to go to Qingdao to bring him back. When I entered the kindergarten, the child-care worker told the kids to call me auntie. "Auntie!" all the kids yelled, and so did Xianping, who couldn't recognize me after my many months' absence. During his stay in the kindergarten, I took a leave once to visit him and another time saw him by chance when I attended a meeting in Qingdao. Wende also visited him while on a business trip. Xianping was consumed by a very high fever, which was soon followed by a blotchy, red rash, starting on his forehead, and eventually spreading over his entire body all the way to his feet. A vaccine for measles was unavailable at that time. The disease was prevalent all year round, and became an epidemic about every three years.

"Mom, I have to go poo," Xianping said. Because his intestines were infected due to the measles he went to the bathroom quite frequently. Diarrhea is one of the common complications of the measles. Every time I put him to bed, he would want to go again. I could hardly get a wink of sleep at night. To further complicate his illness, he soon developed a middle-ear infection that required penicillin shots. Xianping never usually swore at people, but he hated the needles so much that he called the doctor terrible names. He recovered from the measles, but ever since then, he has had a slight hearing problem.

After Xianping got over his measles, my second son, Bingbing, contracted the disease too, but I couldn't take time off and was told not to put my personal interests first. "You just took a leave when your older son was sick weeks ago. It's just measles, no big deal," the hospital president, Ding, said to me. In March, Bingbing's condition worsened. I wanted to take him to a bigger and better hospital, but Ding refused to give me a leave. "Many children have measles, why is your kid so important?" he said to me.

On that fateful night, Wende and I sat silently beside the child's bed. Wende had a gloomy look on his face. Huge sores had broken out on his lips due to anxiety. The old babysitter was settled by a table doing some sewing, stopping to sigh occasionally.

"I should take Bingbing to a better hospital. The resources are limited here," I said to Wende.

"You can't leave without the leader's permission; we don't want to cause trouble," Wende said to me.

"What are we going to do?" I replied angrily, not because I thought that what he said was wrong, but because of my frustration of not having any other options in the matter. I looked at my child with deep worry. He was so small and vulnerable, his little body covered with the red blotchy rash.

It was a very calm night, with no wind at all. Bang! Suddenly the door opened and slammed against the wall, as if someone had broken in. The old babysitter's eyes widened in alarm, and she trembled fearfully. I quickly jumped up to close the door and saw a neighbor just coming home. Since then I have never stopped wondering how the door could have opened by itself, without any wind. I tried to break it down logically. It could have had something to do with the neighbor's door, I reasoned, but was not completely sure. That incident became yet another mystery in our family history.

"It looks like your Bingbing's illness is fatal," the old babysitter said to me at that moment, her voice shaking.

"What makes you say things like that? Not that old superstitious stuff again." I got very upset.

"It's his fate," the old nanny said. "Maybe I shouldn't say this, but the door couldn't open by itself. It was them. They came to take him away."

I understood what she meant by "them" — the demons who were sent by the ruler of the underworld.

"Your elder son, Xianping, has tiger's teeth and does not tolerate any child that is too close to his age. Your children have to be many years apart," the old nanny said in her heavy Shangdong accent.

"Enough of that superstition," I said.

I was angry, not because I considered what she said to be nonsense, but because I was afraid that there could be some truth in the old woman's words. Xianping was sleeping soundly, unaware of what was going on around him. I had never even noticed that the child had "tiger's teeth." Now that the old babysitter had mentioned it, I realized she was right. When he smiled, the long protruding teeth near the front were exposed. I sat anxiously by Bingbing's bed the whole night, thinking about what the babysitter had said.

Three days later, Bingbing had developed the serious complications of pneumonia and encephalitis — inflammation of the brain. Without the leader's permission, I left my work and carried the weak baby to several hospitals. I ended up at the Second Hospital of the 67 Army in Jiaoxian County.

Bingbing died at about eight o'clock in the evening, similar to the time he was born. The Second Hospital would always hold special meaning for me as the place where my first son Xianping was born, and where my second son Bingbing died.

Grief stricken, Wende took Bingbing to the suburbs for a secret burial. There was no coffin, no ceremony. The baby was only wrapped with cloth and buried hastily. This is unimaginable in Western society, but it was a very common practice in China in those days. Burial of the dead was forbidden at the time. According to old customs, a child at that age didn't deserve a coffin. Since Confucius' social order was *jun chen, fu, zi* — ruler, subjects, father, son — children ranked at the bottom and were the least important. Wende didn't want me to go, afraid that I would have a breakdown, so I never did know the exact spot Bingbing was buried.

"I wish I had taken him to a better hospital much earlier — he wouldn't have died," I said to Wende when he came back after the burial.

"It's not your fault. You've done everything you can," he said.

"You can treat the disease, but you can't cure the fate," the old nanny said. "It wasn't a coincidence that Bingbing's illness was passed on to him by his older brother."

Bingbing was such a peculiar child. He started talking at a very early age. He used to point at Wende's military uniform and say "Papa," then point at my white coat and say "Mama." He was quite the opposite of his older brother. Xianping liked apples; Bingbing loved pears. He liked to eat anything that Xianping didn't care for, and never fought with his older brother over food.

"The Great Leap Forward has taken Bingbing away," Wende said sadly. That was the first time I heard him speak negatively about the party's policy.

"You see, her son died anyway even though she took him to other hospitals," President Ding commented after he heard the news that my son had died. Not only didn't he say anything to comfort me, but he criticized me for leaving work without his permission. It reminded me of that old Chinese proverb: "Tyranny is fiercer than a tiger." Confucius was passing through the foot of Mount Tai and saw a woman wailing mournfully beside a grave. He sent his student, Zilu, to investigate. Zilu asked: "Why are you so heartbroken?" The woman said to him: "My father-in-law was eaten by a tiger, my husband was eaten by a tiger, now my son was eaten by a tiger." Zilu asked: "Why don't you leave here?" The woman answered: "There's no tyranny here." Confucius said to his students: "Remember, Tyranny is fiercer than a tiger."

11

THE YEAR OF THE RAT (1960)

AFTER BINGBING DIED, I wanted the babysitter to stay with us in case we had another child. It was not any easy task to find such a good babysitter. She continued to live with us for another two months until gossip started at the hospital.

"I think we have to let the babysitter go. People are gossiping. They say the army officer's wife has a babysitter," Wende said to me. He yielded to the pressure.

"Why do we care what they say?" I said.

At about the same time, the old babysitter's son had a baby and he wanted her to go home to take care of her grandson. So she went back, and I didn't hear from her for a long time.

A few months later, the old babysitter showed up at the door. "My son got TB and needs some antibiotics immediately," she said to me. "I heard it's a real wonder drug. One shot in the butt, the dying person will be up and walking."

"Streptomycin is in short supply," I told her. "But don't worry, I'll somehow manage to get some for you. Just stay with us for a few days." I managed to locate ten bottles of streptomycin for her as soon as possible. Doctors still needed ration coupons for prescribing the drug to their patients, but the supply was better than two years before. That was the advantage of being a doctor. She stayed for several days before heading home with the wonder drug. Only a few months later, she returned. Her son had died.

"My daughter-in-law wanted to get remarried. But I told her not to," the old nanny said to me. "'You have to be chaste to your dead husband,' I said to her. 'Look at me, I was widowed when I was nineteen, and never married again. You have to accept your fate.'"

"You and your old thought," I said. "In our new society, people have a say in who they want to marry. You can't interfere."

"'If you do get married,' I said to her, 'your late husband will haunt you, and you will never have peace in your life. The worst thing is that when you die, your two husbands in hell will fight over you, and cut you in half.'"

Superstition again.

"'Besides,' I said, 'you have a one-year-old son, and no one will marry a widow with a child.'"

I knew the purpose of the old nanny's visit. She needed my help desperately but she was hesitant to ask. Her whole family was starving.

"The whole village is starving. People have started to eat grass, tree leaves, and bark since last fall. Frogs, birds, and grasshoppers, even rats have been eaten. Now it is the worst time ever — there's nothing left," she said. "Some folks were just working in the field, holding ploughs when they suddenly fell to the ground and died."

"Those deaths were probably caused by low blood sugar. At that time, even some water with a little bit of sugar would have saved their lives," I said. "Here's not so good either. Everyone has to go to bed at five o'clock in the evening to save energy."

When the old babysitter departed, I gave her some money and food to take with her. The old lady was moved to tears.

"Doctor Li, I won't be able to repay you for your kindness in this life. Next life, I will be reincarnated into a cow or horse and work hard for you," she said.

"It's the best I can do. Just come when you need help," I said to her.

From 1958 to 1959 during the Great Leap Forward movement, peasants concentrated on making steel and neglected
the crops, leading to declines in agricultural production. To
make things worse, local authorities frequently reported grossly
exaggerated production numbers, which covered the fact for
years. Crops in the field were all rotten because no one took the
time to harvest them. Farming tools like ploughshares and picks
were melted down for steel. During those two years, peasants
were encouraged to eat as much as they wanted, at no cost, in
the public canteen, so by the winter of 1958, the granaries were
empty. Soon the famine became widely spread throughout the
country. In the meantime, Mao continued to export grain to
North Korea and North Vietnam to save face with the outside
world. He also exported grain to the Soviet Union in exchange
for military technology, including nuclear bombs.

According to various sources, the death toll due to famine
was as high as 30 million, the majority being peasants. In some
areas of the countryside, desperate people resorted to cannibalism to stay alive. Throughout history, famine had
periodically wiped out the population by millions, and earned
China a reputation as "the land of famine." Cannibalism was
common during times like this. Lu Xun, the renowned Chinese
writer, once declared that the words "human eating" were
written all over Chinese history. He meant both literally and
figuratively. Peasants played a crucial role in the Civil War
against the Nationalists. Unlike the Soviet Revolution that succeeded first in the urban areas during the late twenties, Mao
believed that the Chinese Revolution could only rely on the
peasants, the majority of the nation's population. Since Mao
himself was born to a peasant family, he used this background
as an advantage to gain the peasants' trust and make them his
most loyal followers. He then betrayed them in the most horrible way one could imagine.

The government blamed it on "bad weather," and the withdrawal of Soviet technical and financial support. The relations

between China and the Soviet Union became deeply strained after the new Soviet leader Khrushchev denounced Stalin. Mao accused the Soviet leadership of deviating from Marxist-Leninism, and of becoming revisionists. After Stalin died, Mao considered himself the leader of the world's Communist movement, and started to promote Maoism. The final collapse of the relationship came in mid 1959 to mid 1960, when the Soviets withdrew all of their technicians and experts, and disrupted many industrial and military projects including nuclear weapons programs. The "free" Soviet aid came at a grave cost. At the depth of the famine, China had to ship grain and meat to the Soviet Union to pay off the debt. Even though the Sino-Soviet split might have contributed to some extent, by and large this great famine was caused by Mao's policy. The "bad weather" was the most ridiculous claim. The weather where we lived was normal in those three years. Even if there was bad weather somewhere, it couldn't have been nationwide.

During a Central Committee plenum in December 1958, Mao, who was mainly responsible for the Great Leap Forward disaster, stepped down from his position as state chairman, but remained chairman of the Communist Party. For the next few years, he stayed on the political sidelines and in semi-seclusion. The National People's Congress elected grim-faced Liu Shaoqi as Mao's successor.

There was only one person who stood up to Mao during the Great Leap Forward. He was Marshal Peng Dehuai, one of Mao's old comrades who played an important role in the Long March, the Anti-Japanese War, the Civil War, and the Korean War. He was known for speaking bluntly and acting on impulse. Peng confronted Mao during the Lushan Conference in 1959, and stated that during the Great Leap Forward disaster "the loss outweighed the gain." Mao immediately removed him from his post as minister of defense and replaced him with Lin Biao. This confrontation with Mao would cost Peng his life during the Cultural Revolution.

In private, Liu Shaoqi attributed the famine calamity to "thirty percent natural disaster and seventy percent man-made," indicating Mao's responsibility. I heard that on one occasion Mao commented about the deaths due to the famine: "Sacrifices can't be avoided if we struggle for Communism. People die every day." Lin Biao echoed him: "So what if some people died? We are a big country." Mao forbid party officials to discuss the "nonsense" of death from starvation. Those who did met severe consequences. Liu paid the ultimate price a few years later.

In the spring of 1960, the hospital sent me to Qingdao City to study the technique of X-raying. Textiles were a major industry in Qingdao and they had their own hospital called Qingdao Textile Worker's Hospital. I was already about three months pregnant. I wore protective overalls made of lead to prevent me from exposing myself to harmful X-rays. There were two kinds of protective clothes in the department — lead overalls or an apron. I always scrambled for the overalls because they covered the whole body.

My teacher Dr. Wang was very surprised to find out later that I was pregnant, and didn't think I should be anywhere near the X-ray Department. He was a good teacher, but didn't talk much, and often look depressed and distracted. After we had gotten to know each other better, he told me that his wife was assigned to work in Xinjiang Province, far in the northwest. He hadn't seen her for almost a year and missed her very much. He couldn't eat or sleep well. They had been married for just one year but had lived together for less than a month. Long-distance phone calls were not available there and even if they were, it would cost a one-month wage to make even a brief call. It usually took more than twenty days for a letter to reach the other end of the country.

This kind of separation was very common. People were told to put "revolution" before their own personal happiness. Transfer to a different place was virtually impossible unless you had connections with officials. Because of the long-term separation, sometimes adultery occurred, and it was a very serious crime in those days. Dr. Wang tried many times to have his wife transferred to Qingdao, or to get himself transferred to Xinjiang to be with her. He went though numerous bureaucratic apparatuses and a lot of frustration, but still didn't succeed. He compared their relationship to "the Herd-Boy and the Weaving Girl" — two lovers in Chinese folklore, who are forcibly separated by the Queen Mother who draws the River of Heaven between them, and they are permitted to meet only once a year, on the seventh day of the seventh lunar month, when tens of thousands of magpies form a long bridge for them to pass over the barrier to reunite.

"Why don't you go there to visit her?" I said. I felt very sympathetic toward him.

"I tried many times, but couldn't get a leave," he said. "I'm the only X-ray technician here."

"Why don't I take your place for a month?"

"Would you do that for me?" he said. I had never seen him so happy. However, it was very difficult for him to bring the matter up again in front of the leaders, so he wanted me to ask on his behalf. I understood his situation, and went to talk to the official in charge of the Political Department. I tried hard to convince him that I had already grasped the skills needed to replace Dr. Wang. At first he was skeptical that I could learn so quickly, then I told him that I already had quite a bit of knowledge about X-rays before I came. He was finally moved by my sincerity, and granted a one-month leave for Dr. Wang. When Dr. Wang heard the good news, he couldn't stop thanking me, and immediately started to plan his trip. A round trip to Xinjiang would take more than one week on the train alone, so in reality, he would have less than three weeks to be with his wife.

Twenty days after I took over from Dr. Wang, my hospital sent me a letter, wanting me to go back to perform X-rays for new army recruits. So I went back before the scheduled length of study.

In July of 1960, Wende received permission from the army to go back to his hometown in Hebei Province to visit his family. They had been writing letters asking for money. He was worried about their situation in the countryside.

"The whole village is starving," Wende said to me upon returning home. He looked exhausted from the long trip. He told me that the funny thing was when the villagers greeted each other with the conventional "Have you eaten?" they would always respond with "yes," though, in fact, they hadn't eaten for days. Villagers possessed a strong desire to keep face, and going hungry was shameful.

"My brother has arthritis," Wende said. "He often went to the pond on the west side of the village at night to catch frogs to eat, staying in the cold water until the early hours of the morning. Now he often experiences severe pain in his back and legs."

"Rumor has it that millions of people have died of hunger, and, in some areas, people ate people to stay alive," I said. "But in the hospital staff meeting, leaders warned the doctors not to discuss the deaths caused by hunger, as it will be considered a crime. Although, they admit that there are many unnatural deaths, and an epidemic disease officially called swelling disease. It's not an actual disease itself, but a symptom of malnutrition. Everyone knows what's been going on, but no one dares to say anything."

"Just don't you say anything," he said.

"So I just pretend I don't know anything?" I asked.

"What can you do? It won't make a difference. Only get yourself into trouble," he said.

The "swelling disease" was nothing new to me. In medical terms, it is called edema — swelling of parts of the body due to accumulation of excess fluid. I had seen many patients come in with the problem. Four doctors worked in the Department of Internal Medicine and we would see about forty to fifty patients a day. Among these patients, more than half suffered from "swelling disease," and most of them came from the countryside. The swelling usually started in the feet, then spread to the knees and eventually through the whole body as the condition got progressively worse. Often the problem became worse when the patients drank water and ate salted vegetables, such as pickled turnip, the most readily available food source. Salt aggravated the condition. During that period, I was allotted a certain amount of sugar every month. People needed ration coupons to buy sugar at the time. I often mixed the sugar with some water and let patients drink. It was better than any medicine I could give them.

In the summer of 1960, I had treated an old couple from the countryside who had the "swelling disease." The old peasant pushed his sick wife to the hospital on a one-wheeled cart. It was a common mode of transportation for the peasants in the Shandong Peninsula. They could balance the one-wheeled cars quite well. During the Civil War against the Nationalists, it was these peasants who risked their lives and pushed the same kind of carts to deliver supplies to the Communist army on the frontline.

When the old peasant arrived at the hospital, he fainted, and the first thing I had to do was to revive him. After I pressed a finger against the old man's skin for a few seconds, it made an indentation due to accumulation of excess fluid. I mixed some water with sugar and let the old couple drink it. A few minutes later, the old man came back to life.

The peasant's wife also had "swelling disease," in addition to an infection in her stomach. She had slept on a *kong* bed mat that was woven from cornstalks. Her swelling stomach was

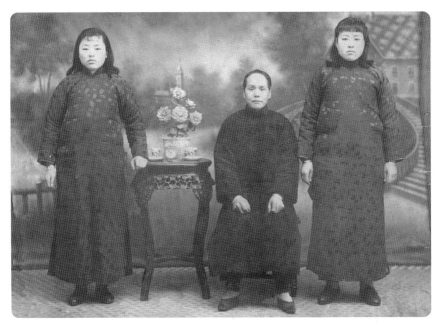

My mother (middle) and me (right) in 1942, a year before she passed away. Chifeng, Inner-Mongolia. This long-lost family photo was discovered by investigators during the Cultural Revolution when my husband and I were persecuted.

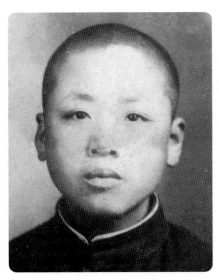

A childhood photo of Wende.

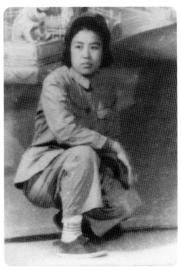

Taken in 1948, in the Northeast, a few years after I joined the Communist Eighth Route Army. I was just starting to study medicine in the Second Regiment of the 13th Brigade.

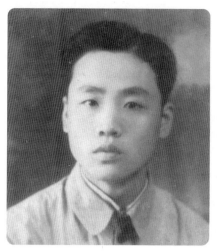

A photo of my late husband Han Wende, taken in 1949. This was the photo he gave to me as a keepsake before entering the Korean War in 1951. Since the military operation was highly secretive, the bottom of his photo, which displayed the "Chinese People's Liberation Army," had to be cut off.

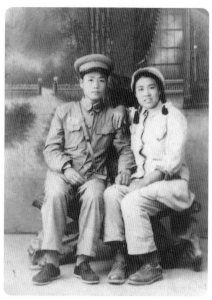

This picture was taken in 1950, when we first met. Changli, Hebei Province.

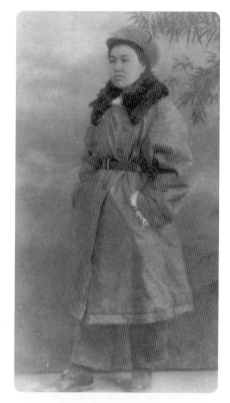

Taken in the Northeast in early 1951 before entering the Korean War. I was wearing an army winter overcoat.

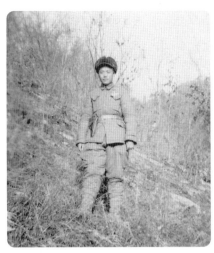

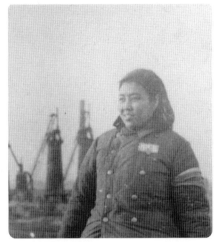

Wende in the winter of 1952 during the Korean War. He was wearing riding britches. North Korea.

In March 1952 during the "Three-Anti's" campaign, when I was called back to China from the Korean battlefield. I was on duty patrolling the concentration camp, which was set up beside an abandoned steel factory. I was wearing the Chinese Volunteer Army uniform with a yellow armband. Tangshan, Hebei Province.

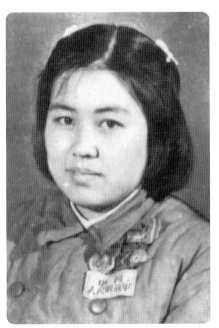

Taken in 1954. I was wearing souvenir badges of the Civil War: the Northeast campaign, Huai Hai campaign and the War of Liberation. The I.D. badge says: Chinese People's Liberation Army.

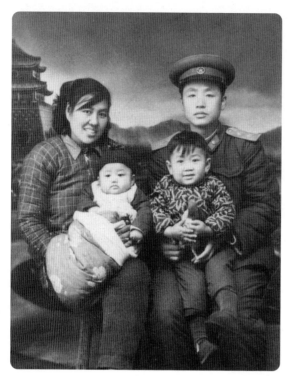

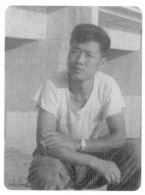

Wende in 1958, during the Great Leap Forward Movement when he was sent to help build a bridge in Jiangsu Province. The photo was taken after the construction was completed.

A family photo taken in the beginning of 1958, the year of the Great Leap Forward Movement. My son Xianping (front right) was three years old, carrying a pigeon in his hands. My second son Bingbing (front left), who died in March 1959, was only three months old. Jiaonan, Shandong Province.

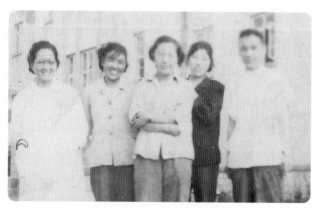

Among colleagues (second from the left) in 1958, during the Great Leap Forward Movement. The photo was taken in front of the Jiaonan County People's Hospital, Shandong Province. There was only one doctor on duty and the rest were doing "voluntary labor" nearby.

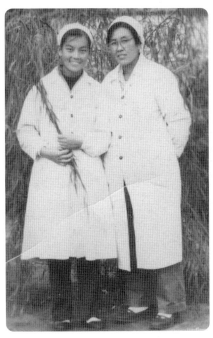

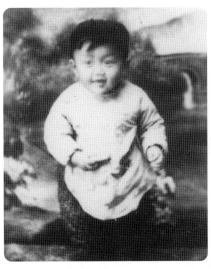

Bingbing in 1958. Jiaonan, Shandong Province. The Great Leap Forward took away his life.

Me (right) with a colleague in 1960s. Jiaonan County Hospital, Shandong Province.

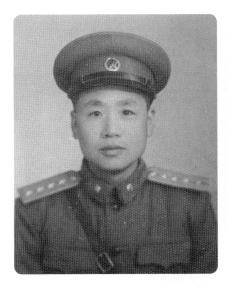

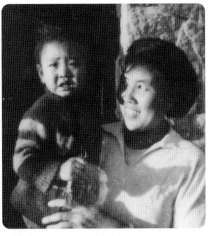

Wende in 1960, when he was promoted to captain. The system of military ranking started in 1955 and was modeled after the Soviet styles. Jiaonan, Shandong Province.

I was carrying my daughter Yanping who was about two years old in 1963. She just went outside the army camp and pulled some of the peasants' wheat. She was crying after I stopped her, still grabbing some wheat in her hand. Jiaonan, Shandong Province.

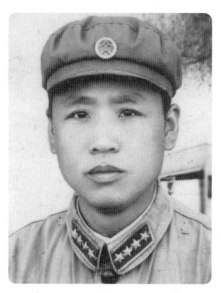

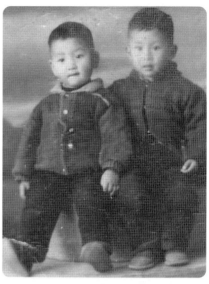

Wende in 1960s. Exact time and location unknown.

My son Luping (left), at about three, with a little friend. Jiaonan, Shandong Province.

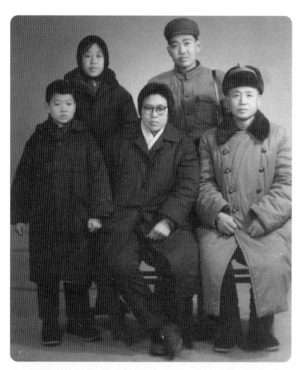

A rare family photo taken in December of 1973, when we just got out of the countryside after we were rehabilitated. Jiaoxian, Shandong Province.

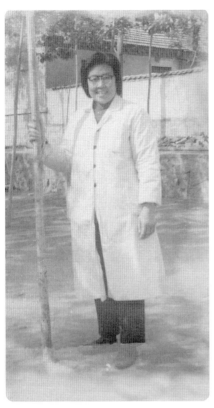

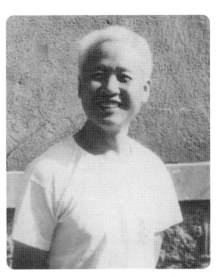

One of Wende's last pictures taken in 1975. Dachang, Shandong Province. The Cultural Revolution took a heavy toll on his health, and consequently led to his death.

Taken in 1975, in the front yard of our residential compound. In the background are hospital wards. Dachang, Shandong Province.

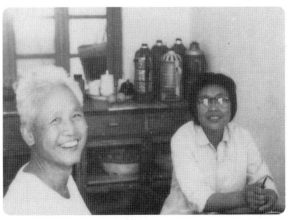

Wende and I in 1979. Dachang, Shandong Province.

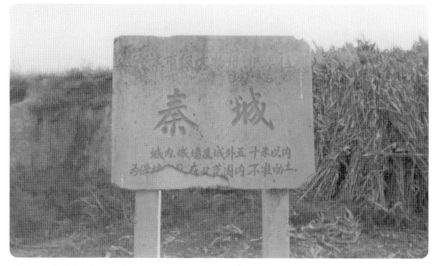

The site of the legendary ancient "Qin City," where villagers believed that treasure was buried. The sign says: The historical and cultural site under the protection of Tinjin city; Qin City; Do not break ground inside the city, on the wall or within fifty meters outside the city. Villagers piled sorghum stalks nearby.

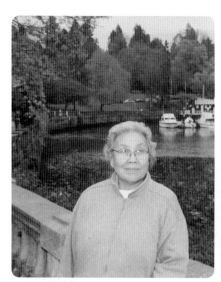

Taken during my visit to Vancouver, Canada, in the fall of 2001. Stanley Park.

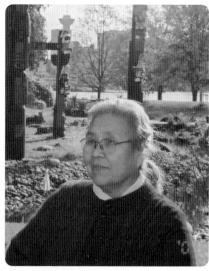

Stanley Park, Vancouver, Canada. 2001.

pierced by a sharp protruding stalk, became infected, and released a terrible odor. Because the tissue under the skin retained an abnormal amount of fluid due to her "swelling disease," the wound was not healing. After the "treatment," I sent both of them home. I also paid the medical fee for them because they didn't have any money.

"We should thank the doctor," the old woman said. "She saved our lives and paid the fee for us."

"Why do we thank her? They have money. They live off the sweat and blood of us peasants," the old peasant said.

The peasants held a great hatred toward anyone who "ate government's grain," as they put it. After so many years of revolution, I was surprised to see this kind of ungrateful behavior from the very people we had fought and sacrificed for. Jiaonan County was one of the earliest liberated areas, but also the poorest. All year round the peasants ate primarily sweet potato chips, which usually became moldy due to long storage in the humid air of the Shandong Peninsula. In fact, the chips often became moldy before being stored because the sweet potato harvest was in the rainy fall season, and the chips wouldn't dry in time. In their attempt to dry the potato chips, the peasants would in desperation use their *kong* beds.

To make things worse, local officials often exaggerated the production output to show their achievements. Even if there was a crop failure that year, the amount of the tax grain delivered to the state would remain the same — and sometimes even exceed the quota. The best grain would be handed to the government and the moldy sweet potato chips left for the people. The peasants had to consume the chips conservatively in order to make them last until the next sweet potato harvest season. Of course, that was before the Great Leap Forward. Now they were lucky if they had moldy chips to eat.

It was at that time when the hospital started to treat patients with *kang fu san* — recovery powder. The ingredients consisted of one pound of ground wheat husk and a half pound of white sugar, which were packed in a plain paper medicine bag. It was a genuine miracle drug and took effect immediately after taking it. The patients would at once come back to life. But even the wonder drug had its shortcomings — its effect was short-lived.

Doctors and nurses in the hospital had tightened their belts up another notch. They often stole carrots in the field on the north side of the hospital when they worked night shift. Whenever a woman was having a baby, doctors would go to the delivery room to ask for placentas, which were supposed to be very nutritious. Dried placenta powder was stored in medicine cabinets at the hospital to be used as a traditional remedy for many diseases. During those dismal years, not as many women as before were having babies, bringing about a dramatic drop in the birth rate. Sometimes, babies were abandoned at the hospital because mothers didn't have the milk to feed them or the means to raise them.

At the same time, the third floor of the hospital ward was reserved for high-ranking cadres. Commissar Feng had checked in a few weeks earlier for a minor health problem. He had left the army and become an important official in the county party committee. Even though he was transferred to the local government, people still respectfully addressed him as Commissar Feng.

The senior-cadre patients would play cards all morning, and, at dinnertime, the cooks would bring up steaming plates of dumplings. The white flour skins were almost transparent and you could see the green chives and meat inside. The doctors, nurses, and patients from below the third floor just stared, mouths watering at the tempting sight. No wonder they said it was paradise upstairs and hell downstairs.

A few days before the Moon Festival, I met up with Dr. Chen who was pacing up and down in the hospital canteen. After operating non-stop for six hours on an important official, he came out of the operating room exhausted and hungry. He had been sent down to the countryside to do manual labor after he was branded as a rightist, and was only now called back to the hospital when an important official needed surgery and was unable to locate a competent surgeon.

Dr. Chen had come to the canteen with a bowl in his hand but he had run out of his food ration for the month. He noticed that the cooks were preparing dumplings for important patients and asked for some of the milky looking water that had been used to boil the dumplings. In that way he thought he didn't have to pay for it.

"The dumpling water will be saved to feed the pigs," the cook said to him.

I felt sorry for Dr. Chen and lent him some food rations. "Big sister," he said to me. He was much younger than I was. "It's very kind of you. I'll pay you back next month when I get my food rations."

"Don't worry about it," I said to him. "I'll get by."

In lunar mid-August, during the Moon Festival, every child in Xianping's kindergarten was given two moon cakes. He eagerly ate one on the bus and had the other one when he got home. At the time, he had already left the Red Star Kindergarten in Qingdao and attended a kindergarten set up by the 201 Division nearby. In the most difficult times, soldiers in 201 Division each saved a 50-gram food ration a day for the children in the kindergarten. The only thing the children ate was porridge — a mixture of pumpkin and millet. Xianping often came home hungry.

In the evening, Wende and I went to watch a war movie called *Fighting North and South*, a Civil War story, specially put on for the officers and their families. We left Xianping at home. The officers, soldiers, and their families filled the large hall to capacity. The soldiers were singing one army song after another before the show started. During the movies the women were very noisy, talking non-stop, because most of them couldn't follow the story. The movie was in progress for only half an hour when the show was interrupted by several loud gunshots outside. All the soldiers immediately jumped up from their seats and rushed out to assemble.

"Spies! Spies!" someone shouted.

"Spies from Taiwan!"

During that time, there were rumors circulating that the Nationalist army was launching a counterattack on the Mainland, because Chiang Kai-shek was convinced that there was famine, and believed that the suffering people would welcome him back. The troop was sent out without delay to search for the spies. Wende and I were ordered to stay and calm down the screaming wives and children of the officials. Traditionally families got together for the Moon Festival. The women were mostly housewives. They were from all over the country so they shouted in many different accents like a bunch of clucking hens roaming helter-skelter in their coop.

The moon was glowing big and round in the clear night sky. Wende and I were bathed in radiant light. A cool breeze touched our faces. It reminded me of that first day when we had met. It had also been on the Moon Festival. But that night, no one was in the mood to appreciate the magnificent full moon. A few hours later, the troop returned empty-handed. The officials commended Wende and me for taking such good care of their families. It was too late to resume the movie after all the commotion.

"My stomach hurts," Xianping said when we arrived back home.

"You probably ate too many moon cakes. You haven't eaten so much at once for such a long time. That's why you feel bloated," I said to him.

I rubbed his aching stomach for a couple of hours until he threw up. From then on, he hated moon cake.

12

"Where Are You, Dr. Li?"

In September of 1960, the Year of the Rat, I was nine months' pregnant. At that time, Wende was at Haiyang, a place situated in the suburbs of Qingdao. The army was digging a tunnel into the mountains in preparation for the imminent war with the Nationalists. They were still using blueprints provided by the Soviet Union, since the work took place before the two countries broke off. Wende worked there for less than one year in the three-mile-long tunnel, which contained electrical power and telephones.

Soon to give birth, I decided to join Wende a hundred miles away. I was hesitant for some time because I was afraid to have the baby on the road. But for some reason, I decided to make the journey, thinking that there would be some hospitals on the way if the unexpected happened. Luckily, the trip went smoothly.

Upon my arrival, I ate lunch, then headed to the local hospital. At five o'clock in the afternoon, I delivered a baby girl. We called her Yanping, a typical girl's name that held no special meaning. According to astrology, she was born under the sign of the rat, and for some reason this would influence her later on.

Only six months after the baby was born, I found myself with a soaring fever of forty degrees and stabbing chest pain on the left, frequently made worse by deep breathing and coughing. I was hospitalized the second day. For ten days, I lay in bed only on my right side without knowing the cause. Wende came into the hospital ward with the six-month-old baby. Afraid of passing the disease on to the baby, I had to stop breast-feeding. The baby hadn't been fed yet and was crying. As soon as Wende stepped one foot outside the ward with the baby in his arms, his eyes filled with tears.

On the tenth day, I was sent to a hospital in Qingdao, where I was diagnosed with pleurisy after fluid was found to have accumulated in my chest. Pleurisy is an inflammation of the thin layers of tissue — pleura — covering the lungs and the chest wall. The condition can make breathing extremely painful, and is sometimes associated with another condition called pleural effusion where excess fluid fills the area between the membrane's layers. The most common cause is viral infection. Other diseases that can cause pleurisy are lung infections such as pneumonia, tuberculosis, and rheumatoid arthritis. Since I was also diagnosed with TB at the time, the doctors weren't sure if the pleurisy had developed from tuber- culosis or rheumatoid arthritis, which I was also suffering, so they treated me for both diseases. This very commonly used method of treatment was called "complete encircling treat- ment." I was treated with streptomycin, penicillin, and many other drugs at the same time.

I had contracted the disease from my patients. Since I had attended the class on continued studies on pulmonary tubercu- losis treatment and prevention, I had more frequent contact with the TB patients at the X-ray Department and at the wards. Even though I always used a sixteen-layered mask, it still didn't prevent me from catching the disease. The average masks used in the hospital consisted of at least eight layers. However, since the masks had to be reused, they carried the risk of being contami- nated if not sanitized properly. To kill the TB bacteria, the masks had to be boiled for at least five minutes. During that period of time, two nurses and a head nurse had also contracted TB from the patients. I stayed in the hospital for two months before recov- ering. The process was slow partly due to malnutrition.

After getting better from pleurisy, my insomnia returned. No sleeping medication worked. I asked for a one-month sick leave and went to Wende's army camp to recuperate. I decided to fight back against the insomnia. Every morning I climbed the mountain nearby, hoping that it would make me extremely tired so I could have a good sleep. It didn't work at all. In fact, the situation became worse because my body was tired but my mind was still very active at bedtime.

To my surprise, I learned later that soldiers had been keeping an eye on me. They noticed that I made my way to the top of the mountain every morning, and suspected that I might be the spy they were searching for. So it seemed that they had been following me diligently for a couple of weeks already. Finally Wende's old comrade Shouyi recognized me. "It's Wende's wife. We are old comrades," he told the soldiers.

Two weeks after I returned to my apartment at the hospital, I was woken up by strange noises at night.

"Did you hear that?" I asked Wende.

"Hear what?" He was half asleep.

"Listen. I think there are rats in the house."

Frustrated, I threw a shoe at them to scare them away. They became quiet for a while. A few seconds later, they came back, repeating the same routine all over again. I threw another shoe. For a long while, the noise didn't reoccur and I thought that the rats had finally learned their lesson. Before I could even finish my thought, they showed up again as if nothing had happened. I got the impression that the rats were purposely irritating me.

I lay in bed with my eyes wide open. It was a familiar and unmistakable feeling. The insomnia had returned, worse than ever. I got up and took some sleeping pills, but they didn't work. I relived my entire life from my childhood all the way to the present. The night became long and exhausting. The baby cried.

"Why does the baby cry so often at night?" Wende said.

I got up, carried the baby, and walked back and forth. "I think she cries at night because I stopped breast-feeding her too abruptly," I said.

"What choice did you have? You didn't want to pass the disease to her."

"I'll make some rice juice for her. Everything is so expensive these days; eggs are seventy cents each."

"We are raising two milk cows on the military farm, and soon she can drink milk," Wende said.

"After I start working in the X-ray Department, I'll have the allowance of two pounds of sugar, five pounds of fish, and five pounds of peanut oil. Do you notice this baby is somehow easier to feed than the other children? She eats anything we give her and is not finicky about food at all," I said.

"What choice do you have when you are born in 1960?"

"I'll go back to work soon and we'll need a babysitter," I said.

I found a woman of about twenty-four to babysit Yanping. My leather shoes and clothes went missing mysteriously. Sugar, which was difficult to come by in those days, ran out very quickly. I finally figured out it was the babysitter who was stealing and I had to let her go.

For three months, I couldn't find a babysitter. At the time, the local armed forces department needed a doctor to examine and evaluate the demobilized soldiers who had various illnesses or injuries in order that medical expenses could be dispensed accordingly. The local armed forces department was a civilian organization that handled the recruitment of new soldiers for the army and the arrangement for demobilized soldiers. The hospital sent me to take care of the job. It was a much lighter job, allowing me to work and watch the baby at the same time. Yanping was quite content in a little cart beside me playing with some toys.

Having been a soldier myself, I had great sympathy for those demobilized servicemen. I always assessed their conditions as being much more serious than they actually were so that they could enjoy better and longer benefits. I determined that one soldier, who had injured his hand and lost a finger, needed to be covered for at least five years of medical expenses. The soldier was so grateful that the following year he presented me with some apples he had grown himself.

A few days after I finished my work at the local armed forces department, the old nanny Sister Liu showed up. She cried when she saw me. "I finally found you, Dr. Li. Where were you? I was looking for you everywhere in the early spring. I wish you were at the hospital that time. Little Stone wouldn't have died," she said.

"Who's Little Stone?"

"My grandson. That poor child. He was all skin and bones when he died. I wouldn't have come to bother you if I could manage, but we had completely run out of things to eat and Little Stone was dying of hunger. I kept calling your name. 'Where are you, Dr. Li, where are you, Dr. Li?'"

"I wish I had been at the hospital at the time," I said.

During the time she described, I had been away from the hospital and studying the technique of X-ray in Qingdao. She had wobbled a long distance on her small bound feet to get there. She hadn't eaten anything for days and had been totally drained of energy.

"I'm looking for Dr. Li," she had asked, not knowing my full name.

"Which Dr. Li?" they had asked.

"The one with glasses," she had said.

"She's not here."

Disappointed, she had dragged herself back home. Her grandson had died days later. I knew that if I had been in the hospital at the time, the child would have made it. Even in the most difficult times, I could have managed to help the family.

"Little Stone, that's a very peculiar name," I said.

"Little Stone, Little Dog — they are all common names for the country boys. It's just a way to cheat the demons. If the kids are worthless, like a stone or an animal, the demons won't bother to take them so they will have a better chance to live," the old nanny said.

Many victims of the famine were children. Children, especially girls, were considered dispensable throughout Chinese history. Ancient records show that neighbors "exchanged their children and ate their bones." Why bones? Because the famine reduced the children to nothing but skin and bones. During times of hunger, children were often sold in exchange for food. Some say about half of those who died during the famine of the early sixties were children under the age of ten.

The old nanny stayed to babysit Yanping. She was the only one I could trust.

After recovering from pleurisy, I had developed severe headaches that no painkiller could cure. In the fall of 1962, after performing two days of X-rays for one thousand new army recruits, my headaches grew increasingly worse, and I felt extremely tired. The blood-test results showed that my white blood cells had been reduced dramatically due to excessive X-ray exposure. I suspected that the headaches had something to do with that too.

In November, accompanied by Wende and my two-year-old daughter, I headed to Beijing to have my headaches checked into. The Xiehe Hospital was very busy. Some patients were waiting to register as early as one o'clock in the morning. When I arrived at the hospital at six, there were already a hundred patients ahead of me. Since I had to go to several departments, it took almost the entire day. In the end, there wasn't even a clear diagnosis.

The next day, after the checkup, Wende and I took Yanping for a tour of the Imperial Palace — also known as the Forbidden City, where emperors once resided and ruled. When we got to the emperor's throne, which was separated from visitors by a rope, Yanping insisted on sitting upon it.

"That's the emperor's throne, it's not for you to sit on," I said.

She kicked, cried, and refused to leave without trying the emperor's throne. At the age of two, she couldn't be reasoned with. Since Wende was wearing the army uniform, the disabled army man watching the site was very sympathetic. He took down the rope and placed Yanping on the throne for a while. There were few people around at that moment. The time that the last emperor, Pu Yi, had sat on the throne might have been short, but Yanping was on it only two minutes before being removed. Nevertheless, she was quite satisfied by the whole thing.

"You are happy now?" Wende said to her.

"How did it feel sitting on the emperor's throne?" I said.

In Beijing, we stayed in a small hotel on Dongzhimenwai Street. There was a stove to keep the room warm. In the morning, just after we checked out and had stepped out of the hotel door, the attendant chased us down. Yanping, who had sat on the emperor's throne just the previous day, had peed on the hotel bed and was fined eighty cents.

When I lay awake at night, I could hear groups of rats running back and forth through the apartment. The rat situation had gotten worse. They showed no signs of fear at all. As soon as the light went out, they would be out. They were very active, chasing each other, and chewing on the wooden bed frames and cupboard. It seemed that when they were in a large group, they felt their behavior was justified, and became very bold.

"We've got to do something about it," I said to Wende.

"We've already tried everything. For over a month they never touched the food on the mousetraps. What a bunch of smart little creatures," he said.

"There has to be something we can do about it. We can give the poison-coated peanuts a try, I heard that they like peanuts," I said.

Yanping suddenly sat straight up in the bed with a stunned look on her face. She went to the bathroom, and, on the way back, stopped in the kitchen for something to eat.

"She's sleepwalking again. It's all because I stopped breast-feeding her too suddenly," I said.

"It's funny she won't remember anything the next day," Wende said.

Yanping went back to bed and ground her teeth in her sleep. It sounded like the rats chewing on the furniture.

"It's definitely an ominous sign," I said to Wende. Once I was awake, there was no way for me to fall back asleep.

Several days passed, and the poison-coated peanuts went untouched. A week later, Yanping was sent to the hospital emergency room. It turned out that she was playing under the bed, ate those poisonous peanuts, and became wildly sick. She was forced to drink a terrible-tasting blue liquid to cleanse her stomach.

"How do you feel now?" the doctor who treated her asked.

"Better," she replied.

"What's your name?" the doctor asked.

"I'm a rat," she said.

"You were born in the year of the rat. I'm asking you what your name is."

"I'm a rat."

The doctors and nurses laughed.

About a month later, the old nanny told me about Yanping's little secret. "Your daughter surely has rat in her," she said.

"What do you mean?" I said.

"She has little rats under the bed."

"Little rats?"

"She is raising several tiny baby rats inside a box under the bed. She feeds them with small pieces of steamed buns."

I found the little hairless creatures all cuddled together. I became upset and threw them out. Yanping was so distraught that she cried for days and refused to eat.

To compensate Yanping for losing her little rats, I got her a cute little chick. She liked it very much. It soon grew up, and was placed into a bigger cardboard box with some holes in it. It was a very pretty chick, pure white with black rings around its eyes. It helped her forget the rats for a while.

At the time, a pregnant woman suffering from anemia arrived at the hospital. Like so many during the early sixties, the woman was malnourished. I advised the woman's husband to cook a chicken for his wife because she needed nutritious food immediately. The next day, Yanping's chicken vanished. She was broken-hearted for several days. A week later, when the pregnant woman's husband was caught stealing, I was informed that he had confessed to stealing chickens throughout the neighborhood, including Yanping's pet.

13

SEEING CHAIRMAN MAO

I BECAME PREGNANT again in the summer of 1963. At the time, there was a family planning policy to control overpopulation, but the policy wasn't strict at all, since Chairman Mao believed "more people, more power." Even though it wasn't such a big deal to have another child, I didn't want anyone to know that I was expecting, afraid that people would gossip. Since I was wearing a doctor's white coat, no one noticed that I was pregnant even up until the last day of my pregnancy. Even during the later stages of pregnancy, I went to work daily and participated in physical labor as usual.

The day before giving birth, I was still painting the hallway of the hospital with my co-workers. "You people paint the top part and I'll paint the bottom part," I said to them, not wanting to get on the ladder in case of an accident.

On a midnight in April in 1964, when I was finally due, I walked into the Obstetrics Department alone. The doctor on duty in the delivery room was the one who had caused several accidents resulting in the deaths of mothers and their babies. However, because she was the wife of an important official, nobody dared to say a word about it. She was originally from Shanghai. Her hands were always oily for some reason, perhaps from constantly touching food and equipment at the same time.

"You'd better get on the bed; you are about to give birth," she said to me.

As I lay on the table worrying, I developed a very ominous feeling about the situation. I was all by myself in the delivery room, since Wende was at the military camp ten miles away and could only come home on Sundays. After midnight, I was so exhausted that I fell asleep on the bed, not waking until six the next morning.

At six-thirty, a very good doctor came on duty. "Thank Chairman Mao for that," I said to myself. "The baby will be born under a lucky star." It was almost as if the baby had known the situation and waited until the next morning to come out.

At seven o'clock, the baby was born. The delivery room was on the east wing of the hospital, so as the sun rose, brilliant sunshine shone upon us. We called him Luping. Lu was short for Shandong Province.

"This boy was born in the year of dragon — it's a very lucky sign," I said to Wende when he came to the hospital. "There's a nurse in the hospital, she had six children, all girls. She asked me if she could switch a girl for our son. They really want a son."

"How could you agree with that?" he said. His face was all red.

"I didn't agree," I said. "Don't be so serious."

There was another colleague of mine whose surname was Liu. She insisted that the baby should wear the little clothes her children had worn before because Liu was pronounced the same as "stay," which meant the baby would survive.

On a hot summer night, four months after Luping was born, I was woken up by some strange sounds. I had poor eyesight but sharp ears. A slight noise could disturb me.

"Did you hear that?" I said to the babysitter.

"No, what is it?" the old woman mumbled, half asleep.

After turning on the light, to my surprise, I saw shoes floating at the side of the bed. It took me some time to realize what was going on. The water was seeping in through the seam of the door and it had risen almost as high as the bed.

"Water!" I yelled.

"Good Heavens! Where's the water coming from?" the babysitter exclaimed.

Luping was sleeping soundly and calmly, completely ignorant of what was happening around him. Shortly I heard people shouting, "Everyone go to the top floor."

Not even having time to find our shoes, I carried Luping; the babysitter grabbed Yanping, and we headed to the fourth floor of the building. It was chaos. Children were crying, and women were screaming hysterically. I lost all my medical books to the flood. They were very expensive to replace. The whole night, we waited on the fourth floor for the water to recede. It had been raining steadily for many days already.

"The year of the dragon has often been disastrous," the old babysitter said. "The dragon king is the ruler of the waters — seas, rivers, and rain clouds. And he's angry now. People must have done something bad and offended him. Luping was born under a very powerful sign."

In the winter of 1965, when Luping was less than two years old, he developed measles, and wasn't allowed to go out. Staying inside all day was a very difficult thing for a child to do. He liked to eat lunch while watching the guinea pigs that the nearby Bureau of Health raised for experimental purposes. He would cry and kick. The old babysitter had to carry him to different places in the house, one moment the kitchen, and next to the bedroom. Every time he was placed in a new spot, he would stop crying temporarily.

It took him twenty days to get over the measles without complications of any sort. Yanping was in the same room with him. Sooner or later she would have measles, I thought, so there was no point in separating them. But she didn't get infected that time. It wasn't until next the year that she had her measles, which also went smoothly.

Wende was promoted from captain to major that year. His position was the head of the supply department of the 601

Regiment, 201 Division, a rank equal to that of a regimental commander. Lin Biao, the Defense Minister abolished all the standard military ranks that same year.

In the several years following the Great Leap Forward fiasco, political movements were seemingly absent. However, the reality couldn't be further from this. Mao unmistakably blamed the famine disaster on sabotage by "class enemies" who intended to restore capitalism. After he stepped down as state chairman, moderates like Chairman Liu Shaoqi and the party's General Secretary Deng Xiaoping started some corrective measures, emphasizing realistic planning rather than seeking instant success. They decentralized the People's Commune by giving more power to the production brigades and teams. Each peasant was allotted a small plot for private use and was also allowed to operate a small part-time business, such as selling chickens and eggs, to earn some extra money. These measures contributed significantly to the economic recovery. While all this was happening, Mao, still holding great power, believed that capitalism was creeping up, and maintained his belief that the main struggle was still between socialism and the capitalism.

In the beginning of 1961, the worst time of the famine, Mao was already playing with the idea of starting some kind of purification campaign to stop anti-socialist tendencies and capitalism from creeping up. The plan was suspended (although not for long) due to the collapse of the economy and the opposition of Chairman Liu Shaoqi and the party's General Secretary Deng Xiaoping. But it didn't stop Mao from bringing the plan up again in 1962 when economic recovery was just underway. In 1963, Mao pushed the political campaign — Four Cleanups — into full bloom. By 1965, under the cover of the Four Cleanups movement, Mao had gradually regained his control of the party with the support of the National Defense Minister Lin Biao, a radical opportunist.

Four Cleanups, also called the Socialist Education movement, started that same year. It addressed problems in politics, economics, organization, and ideology, and it resembled the Three-Anti's movement of 1952 and the Anti-Rightist movement of 1957. But this campaign was smaller-scale, a prelude to a much greater political movement — the notorious Cultural Revolution. Some even compared the Four Cleanups movement to the Yan'an Rectification campaign of 1942–45, which was intended to increase ideological correctness.

Before the movement, Hospital President Ding asked me if I could do him a favor by getting a wash basin from Wende's army store. Those things were very difficult to come by. I bought the item for him. He promised to pay me back the six yuan for the basin but never did. When the Four Cleanups movement started, he accused me of bribery. I put up a poster in the hospital to clear my reputation. Who would have thought something as small as a wash basin could end up having political consequences?

During the movement, a hospital accountant was one of those attacked after being accused of embezzlement. The amount wasn't large, but the charges quickly escalated to an allegation that he was a spy for both America and Taiwan. As a result of such a harsh accusation, he hanged himself.

The movement also dealt with "illicit sexual relations." Any sexual relations outside of marriage were considered illicit. People were encouraged to catch adulterers in the act, so they were always on the lookout. Scouts were rewarded, and the guilty party was punished. Adulterers who were discovered were forced to write a full confession describing their relationships in explicit detail. When they were ordered to publicly read their "self-criticism articles," which contained detailed obscenities, the drowsy crowd would suddenly come back to life after the long boring political meeting and listen with attentiveness and exhilaration.

It was also in 1965 that I was sent down to the countryside with a mobile medical team. In January, Mao approved the Health Ministry's "Report on Sending the Mobile Medical Team to the Countryside." In the first half of the year, close to 30,000 doctors from all over the country made their rounds visiting patients in the rural areas. In June, Mao issued an instruction to "shift the focal point of the medical and health work to the countryside." A decade and a half after the Communists' takeover, the peasants still didn't have access to doctors and medicine. Ninety percent of the well-trained doctors were in the cities, while only ten percent were in the countryside where eighty percent of the population lived. Mao blamed the Health Ministry which was dominated by Western-trained doctors who only served the *laoye* — masters. Rather than trying to provide health care for the peasants, he was more politically motivated, possibly partly to undermine the Health Ministry, or maybe to regain the peasants' trust after the great famine.

In the fall, I was sent down to the remote countryside in Jiaonan County with another woman doctor and two nurses. We stayed in the countryside for over a month and made our rounds in five villages. Four of us, all women, lived in villagers' homes, and ate with them. The main food was steamed corn bread, shaped like cones and hollow in the middle. Occasionally we had homemade tofu — a mixture of boiled vegetables and ground soybeans.

When villagers heard the doctors from the county hospital had come, they all wanted to take advantage of the free consultation and medicine. Among the twenty or thirty patients we saw each day, most were women with gynecological diseases. Another thing that greatly surprised me was that some young girls in the villages were still secretly engaging in the old-fashioned foot-binding tradition. It was as if they had absolutely no contact with the outside world. Surprisingly, I also found many villagers with neurosis — an obsolete, vague term that refers to any mental imbalance. Many women came to see me with depression, anxiety, fear, and other phobias. This was completely out of my scope of practice, and I didn't know where to refer them to. Psychological consultation was unheard of in those days, even in the cities. It was difficult for us to treat even conventional diseases because all we had was a medicine box containing basics such as aspirin. We had to refer the serious patients to the closest hospital. So in a sense, mobile medical teams were a mere political formality that couldn't fundamentally change the medical situation in the countryside, especially considering that the doctors' stay was temporary. More absurdly, some doctors were sent down to the countryside to work in the name of the Four Cleanups campaign — another indication of Mao's political motives for interest in the medical programs.

In the summer of 1966, I was sent by the hospital to perform first aid for people who were swimming in the ocean nearby to show their support for Chairman Mao.

In July, Chairman Mao took his renowned "swim" in the Yangtze River near Wuhan to dispel rumors of his illness. His picture appeared in all the newspapers throughout the country, each one claiming that at the age of seventy-three the chairman could swim faster and further than an Olympic champion. Later we found out that, according to Mao's personal doctor, he didn't really swim, but rather floated downstream on his big stomach. Nonetheless, the news caused a sensation throughout the country. Everyone — men and women, soldiers and civilians — plunged into the water wherever they could find some to show their support of Mao.

I told the officials that I didn't know how to swim but they wouldn't take no for an answer. I had no choice but to get into the water and was almost swept away by the undercurrent. I swallowed several mouthfuls of salty sea water and developed a phobia about water following the event.

Following the calamity of the Great Leap Forward and the great famine, Mao lost a significant amount of power to his rivals, Liu Shaoqi and Deng Xiaoping, and kept a fairly low profile after that. After the successful swim in the Yangtze River, Mao sent a significant signal to the public that he was back in the political front. It marked the start of the Great Cultural Revolution — the first mass action against party leaders at the highest level. This power struggle ultimately touched the lives of nearly every person and brought the country to the brink of civil war. At the time, Mao had been growing further apart from the moderates, who opposed his policies. The party divided into two groups. On the one side were Mao and Lin Biao, supported by the People's Liberation Army (PLA); on the other side were Liu Shaoqi and Deng Xiaoping, who had their strength in the regular party machine.

Mao was convinced that he could no longer depend on the formal party organization, which had been infiltrated by the capitalists and bourgeois. He turned to the one thing he knew best: revolution. Mao called on students to rebel against authority. These young people, initially high-school students, then joined by university students, came to be known as the Red Guard. The Red Guard groups swiftly formed around the country, with millions gathering in Beijing to receive the blessings of their great leader. In the fall, Mao received millions of frantically cheering Red Guards on Tiananmen Square. Standing beside him was second-in-charge, Lin Biao, waving Mao's Little Red Book. During the beginning of the Cultural Revolution, Lin Biao became known as "the dearest and closest comrade of Chairman Mao" and gained a reputation for "the slogan of Long Live Chairman Mao never leaves his mouth; Chairman's Mao's Little Red Book never leaves his hand." He was single-handedly responsible for Mao's cult. He called Mao "our great leader, great teacher, great commander, and great helmsman," which became widely used by average people. Lin was considered a military strategist and a somewhat comic figure in history. He became one of the most prominent generals after he defeated the Japanese in the Battle of Pingxingguan in 1937. A few months later, he wore an overcoat captured from the Japanese and got shot by a Nationalist soldier who mistook him as a Japanese officer. He sustained a severe spinal nerve injury and developed a phobia toward water and light. He was bedridden during the fifties, eating and going to the toilet without leaving bed. Later, according to Mao's personal doctor, Lin's illness was more mental than physical.

Another person who emerged as a powerful political figure during the beginning of the Cultural Revolution was Jiang Qing, commonly known as Madame Mao. She was an actress before she became Mao's fourth wife. She collaborated with Lin Biao and was responsible for inciting the Red Guard against Chairman Liu Shaoqi and Deng Xiaoping. She was also behind the creation of the eight *Yang Ban Xi* — model plays with Communist or revolutionary themes — the few operas and ballets that were permitted during the Cultural Revolution. These soon-put-you-to-sleep plays included *The Legend of the Red Lantern, Shajiabang, Seizing the Tiger Mountain by Strategy*, and the ballet the *Red Detachment of Woman*. She was diagnosed by Mao's personal physician as being a hypochondriac because of her unfounded belief that she was suffering from serious illnesses and her irrational fears of dying. More strangely, she had used eight different names throughout her life.

By reviewing Red Guards in Beijing, Mao had officially set off the most devastating force which spread like a shock wave throughout the country. The young Red Guards went on a nationwide rampage of destruction, known as the "red terror" phase. Millions were publicly humiliated, tortured, and beaten to death. Books were burned, ancient art destroyed, historical sites vandalized, and churches and temples torn down. Soon

Red Guard groups became widely spread. Factories, hospitals, and all other workplaces promptly set up their own Red Guard organizations. Even though the students were still active at this phase, the major role had shifted to the workers who called themselves Rebels — a word that the general public often used interchangeably with the name Red Guards, and sometimes even Red Guards Rebels was used. Soon armed conflicts broke out between the rival Rebel organizations. Rebel organizations evolved from the young Red Guard, but during the two-year armed conflicts between 1967 and 1968, these groups became quite different. Their members were from all walks of life, and their goal was to seize power from the various levels of governments across the country. Some of the Rebels were in fact criminals. An accountant who was under investigation during the Four Cleanups movement ran away from the hospital. When the Cultural Revolution started, he came back, and became one of the Rebel leaders.

In January 1967, Rebels overthrew the Shanghai Party leaders in the so-called January Storm. Soon afterward, many ministries were seized and the nation slid into total anarchy.

It was just before this period, in September 1966, that Yanping started school. In her first class she learned to write "Long live Chairman Mao." Xianping, at eleven, graduated from elementary school and started junior high school at First High School. A few months later, he came home at noon.

"Why have you come home so early?" I asked.

"There's no teacher in my class. Teacher Zhang, who is in charge of my class, has been locked up in the classroom by the students. They said he was a bourgeois academic authority. We have to take turns watching him," he said.

I knew Mr. Zhang quite well. The school was very close to the hospital so it was convenient for Mr. Zhang to sneak by with a lunchbox in his hands to complain about Xianping's behavior in school, and, at the same time, seek medical treatment for his ulcer. He often informed me that Xianping needed to pay more attention in class and study harder. I had told Xianping many times but he never listened.

"In the old days, teachers beat up students, and now it's the opposite." I told Xianping how I was beaten by the teacher with a rattan stick when I was young.

"Oh, I almost forgot. I need some tea," Xianping said.

"What's it for?" I asked.

"It's for Teacher Zhang. He asked me if I could bring him some tea, and I said yes. I feel sorry for him."

"Alright, I'll put some jasmine tea in an envelope," I said. My son was very generous. He often came home begging for money to buy notebooks and pencils. I wondered why they ran out so quickly. Then I found out later that he always gave them away to the poor country kids in his class who couldn't afford them. The country kids used their pencil ends right until they couldn't grab them in their hands.

In late fall, Xianping went on a four-day bus tour with some older schoolmates. He liked to follow those bigger kids around. Exchanging revolutionary experiences, as they called it. I packed a knapsack with some necessities for him, like a water bottle and an army blanket. When Wende came home and found out about it, he was very upset with me.

"How could you let an eleven-year-old kid go on a trip by himself?" he said.

"Don't worry, he's with a group," I said.

"Those are all kids."

"They have more power than we do. When the head of the young Red Guard demands a bus from the bus depot, no one dares to refuse."

"What is he going to eat and where is he going to stay?" Wende said.

"Everywhere they go, there are Red Guard Stations that will provide food and shelter for them. He'll be all right," I said.

When the group returned four days later, Xianping was not amongst them. Wende was furious. "You have spoiled the kid; you let him do whatever he wants," he said.

Xianping came home two weeks later. It turned out that he had stayed with my old friend in Jiaoxian. As soon as he came back from the trip, he wanted to go to Beijing to see Chairman Mao, who was receiving Red Guards in Tiananmen Square.

"No way," I said. "It's too dangerous, I have heard rumors that the crowds in Tiananmen were so large that many kids were injured, even crushed to death."

"But many of my classmates are going," he said.

"I have to discuss it with your father first. I don't think he agrees either."

Xianping sulked for several days. Seeing Chairman Mao was the most honorable thing a person could do in those days. In films I had seen people shouting and crying frantically when they glimpsed Chairman Mao. I told Wende about it when he came home on the weekend. Needless to say, he didn't agree with Xianping going to Beijing.

It was not just kids who were doing that. The adults from the factories and other units would come to the hospital at the time to exchange revolutionary experience. There were even people from Beijing. Even the patients didn't stay in their beds, running about from ward to ward, pushing their intravenous stands. Some of them were more active than the healthy people.

"I heard that the officials in the 201 Division are also planning to go to Beijing in a group to see Chairman Mao. So eventually someone in our family will have the honor of seeing our great leader," Wende said to me.

14

CUTTING PONYTAILS

"LI QUNYING, GET UP and go to receive Chairman Mao's latest instruction," the Red Guard leader shouted at midnight, when I had just managed to get to sleep.

"Immediately!" he added.

Startled, Yanping sat straight up in bed, disoriented as she looked around the room and murmured something I couldn't figure out. Then she lay down and drifted off again.

I got up without delay and headed to the Red Guard head-quarters where everyone received Chairman Mao's Little Red Book. Then we were instructed to write twenty posters before we were allowed return home. I had no idea what to write so I copied some sentences from Chairman Mao's Little Red Book. I knew I couldn't possibly go wrong by doing that.

After finishing several posters, I was completely drained. In the end, I just wrote "Long live Chairman Mao" on every remaining page, muddling through my quota. Then we took the posters to the streets and glued them onto every possible surface: walls, doors, trees, and power poles. The posters that were just put out a few hours earlier were soon covered by new ones from rival factions. The paper on the walls con-tinued to grow, layer by layer, sometimes reaching a thickness of several inches. When I got home, it was already four o'clock in the morning. During those days, I never removed my clothes at night so that when the Red Guards came calling for me, I could just jump out of bed and head out the door.

In our hospital alone there were several Red Guard factions. Red Coat Battle Regiment and Yanan Battle Regiment were the biggest. Smaller groups also existed and they had symbolic names like "The Eagles," "Red Flag," and "Revolutionary Rebels." At first I didn't know which organization to join. However, I knew I had to take part in one of them. I couldn't just sit on the fence. Like they always said: "You are either a revolutionary or a counter-revolutionary." There was nothing in between. The Red Coat Battle Regiment was the faction with the most members and I thought to myself that going with the majority would never be wrong. Besides, the Red Guard leader was working class, and as Marx said: "The working class leads all." He was just a common laborer who worked in the emergency power room and sometimes helped carry corpses to the morgue. Before the Cultural Revolution, no one paid any attention to him. Now he had suddenly become very powerful and everyone, including the hospital leaders, had to listen to him.

When he told me to take down the old pictures of fairy maidens on the walls in our home, I obeyed. Even though these were just traditional New Year pictures, according to him, they were typical Four Olds: old thought, culture, customs, and habits. All those things had to be destroyed. Even my daughter Yanping's ponytails had to be cut off because they were also Four Olds. I had no choice but to cut them off. She had been wearing those two beautiful ponytails since she was two years old. She cried for several days.

Mass Red Guard rallies were frequent during that time. Many doctors, staff, even the hospital officials were publicly denounced, tortured, beaten to death, and driven to suicide. It was common for several different organizations to take turns denouncing one person until midnight, with each session lasting for hours. With so many Red Guard organizations, each one claiming that they represented Chairman Mao's thought and the true spirit of the Cultural Revolution, the hospital soon fell into a complete state of chaos.

A fifty-year-old patient came into the emergency room with acute symptoms, such as severe abdominal pain and distention of the abdomen; one doctor diagnosed that he had intestinal obstruction and required urgent surgery to relieve the blockage. The family members carried the patient upstairs to the operating room on the fourth floor. The surgeon belonged to a different Red Guard organization and didn't think the surgery was necessary; he sent the patient back to the doctor in the emergency room. So the family carried the patient downstairs.

"There's nothing I can do about it," the doctor said. "I'm a physician, not a surgeon. The patient needs surgery at once."

The family struggled to carry the patient upstairs one more time and again the surgeon refused to do the operation. Several hours had passed since the patient first came into the hospital. The family hauled the patient up and down the stairs many times until he died. No one claimed responsibility for the patient's death.

A female factory worker, who had accidentally gotten her hand caught in a machine, came into the emergency room. The first thing a doctor asked was not what had happened to her hand but rather to which faction she belonged. After the doctor found out that she was part of a different faction, he refused to operate on her. She was forced to go to a different hospital where her whole hand had to be amputated because of the delayed surgery.

It was in the first year of the Cultural Revolution that my colleague Dr. Yang, a gynecologist, was driven to suicide by the Red Guard groups. She was one of the few highly educated doctors in the hospital. She was already fifty years old but had never married, and that became her crime. Her fiancé had run away with the Nationalists to Taiwan before liberation. "The old virgin" was denounced in mass rallies many times. "Why aren't you married? Are you waiting for your fiancé? Are you expecting the Nationalists to come back?" they questioned her. Many of the Red Guards who denounced her were her former students. She was very strict with her students. Once, a student had one button missing on her uniform so Dr. Yang ordered her to go back to sew it on before returning to class. Dr. Yang was somewhat eccentric and society couldn't tolerate this. After she hanged herself, her old cat refused to eat and died shortly after.

Staying single was a crime. A forty-year-old woman who worked in a department store came to see me. She had never gotten married. The Red Guards had surrounded her in a circle and pushed her around, demanding that she confess why she was still single at her age. "Are you hiding something?" they said. In the end, she had no choice but to reveal to them that she wet the bed every night and she was ashamed to tell anyone, so she had never got married. The Red Guards all laughed at her. She told me that she had struggled with this problem since she was young. Every night she had to place a piece of plastic underneath her bedsheet, and in the morning she would wash the sheet before her roommates got up.

"Why didn't you come earlier?" I asked.

"I was ashamed of myself before. Now the secret is exposed and everyone knows it, so I have nothing to hide anymore," she said.

"There's nothing to be ashamed of," I said. "I see this all the time. It's very easy to cure."

"Is it?" She was surprised. "I was too embarrassed to see a doctor," she said.

After only a few treatments, she was cured. About a year later, married with a baby, she came back to thank me. "If it wasn't for the Red Guard exposing my problem, I probably would never have gotten married and had a baby," she said. She was very grateful to me and the Red Guard.

Violent conflicts between the different Rebel factions were common. In the spring of 1968, when the Cultural Revolution was in its third year, I was called to examine the Rebel leader's body in the morning. He was dangling from a tree in the yard. With help from two men, we managed to get him down. The body was already still, so I could tell he had been hanging there for a long time already, probably since the night before.

A young Red Guard didn't dare to come near and shouted at me at the top of his lungs while he stood eighty feet away from the scene.

"I order you to rescue him!" he shouted.

I turned around and shouted back at him, "There's nothing I can do, even if you shoot me. He's dead."

I noticed that the rope had left a complete circular mark right around his neck. If he hanged himself, the rope would leave a horseshoe shaped mark, not a complete circle. I suspected that he was strangled with the rope before he was strung up in the tree. Since I had often assisted coroners at work before, I could tell something was fishy.

I had learned some basics from the coroner, a middle-aged male police officer from the county's public security bureau. The bureau needed an assistant from the hospital, and the requirement was that the candidate had to be a trustworthy party member who could keep secrets, and who also was not afraid of corpses. So the hospital chose me for the job. I was qualified for both criteria since I had seen numerous dead bodies on the battlefield, unlike some doctors who were really faint-hearted. Just a few nights earlier, when a patient died in the emergency room, I had to carry the corpse to the morgue with a male doctor. He was scared to death. He wanted me to carry the front end of the stretcher so that he would be the last to enter the morgue and the first to get out. The morgue was a small, detached building with a few concrete platforms inside.

When I opened the door, some sparrows inside were startled and flew out. The doctor dropped the stretcher and ran out of the morgue, his unbuttoned white coat fluttering in the air as if he was a ghost himself.

The coroner came to the hospital once a week to teach me some basic forensics, such as how to tell if a floater was murdered or had committed suicide. Goosebumps on the skin and water in the stomach indicated that the person had drowned, possibly suicide; otherwise it might indicate that the victim had died before being placed in the water — murder. It was a gruesome job, but I couldn't turn it down.

Murder was very common in those lawless days. In the fall of 1968, I assisted a coroner in conducting an autopsy in the suburbs. A peasant had located a body in a reservoir. The body was standing erect at the bottom of the water with a big stone tied to its feet. We had to get divers to recover the body. Two divers, outfitted with heavy, clumsy diving gear, were sent down to handle the grim task. The bloated body had already started to decompose, making it unidentifiable. As the coroner examined the corpse's face with a large set of tweezers, a big chunk of flesh fell away from the cheek, exposing the teeth, which included two gold molars at the back of the mouth.

"Could this be the secretary who disappeared?" I said to the coroner. "He had two gold molars."

At once, everyone remembered a fire that had broken out in the town hall just a few weeks earlier. There was chaos as everyone scurried to extinguish the blaze with basins and buckets. The flames could be seen from miles away. After the fire was finally out, they discovered that the secretary was mysteriously missing.

I remembered that the secretary had come to see me several times about his toothache; I referred him to the best dentist in the hospital and he was very grateful. We called upon the secretary's family to identify the body. Judging from the teeth, they were almost certain it was him. Even though the body was decomposing, the two gold molars still remained intact and sparkled. It seemed as if they were trying to reveal a mystery. There was no investigation being conducted concerning the secretary's death.

During that period, Wende was sent to the local government to "support the leftists," which in reality meant to restrain the leftist radicals and restore order. He and his team attended local staff meetings and the mass rallies. Revolutionary committees were set up in every work unit. These committees, which consisted of unit leaders, army officers, and Red Guards, held power over any other organization.

Wende was apparently worried about the situation. "It's really getting out of control. Everyone is feeling insecure these days. People eat too much and don't know what to do with themselves," he said to me. "Be very careful what you say these days. Remember, don't ever say anything in front of a third person."

"Why is that?" I asked. I knew what he was going to explain it to me, but I asked anyway.

"Because if the other party decides to expose you, he won't be able to find anyone to testify against you."

The same month, I attended a large-scale mass rally against the hospital president, Ding.

A carpenter had discovered by chance that President Ding was going to bed with a young man who worked in the hospital. When the matter was reported to the Hospital Revolution Committee, it caused a huge commotion. The older people all understood the nature of the matter, but the young Red Guards from high school were clueless as to what was going on. Homosexuality was unheard of in those days. Together with another doctor, they brought me into the office to explain the situation. We gave the students a physiology and anatomy lesson. I hated to explain that kind of matter to the young people, but it was necessary for the sake of the revolution. They were finally convinced that it was the truth.

"That dirty son of a bitch! How could he do such a disgusting thing?" The young Red Guards were filled with indignation.

"That's definitely a counter-revolutionary act!"

They became very agitated. "Let's get him!" I finally understood the significant role the young students had played in the revolution: they were full of youthful spirit and revolutionary vigor, and they were quick to act. No wonder that Chairman Mao compared them to "the sun at eight or nine o'clock."

They immediately exhibited posters to expose Ding, and suspended him from his position pending further investigation. President Ding's wife hadn't known what was going on either. She came into the committee office and they cleared things up for her. She felt very embarrassed. "What a shameful thing to do! He has a wife and children. How could he do that?"

Rifling through the documents in his office, they came across more evidence against President Ding. They discovered a secret file that he had kept. Apparently he had taken great effort over the years to develop a system of dividing everyone in the hospital into three main political categories: good, mediocre, and bad. Many people were blacklisted, including me. In my personal file, he had added: "class alien, work under supervision." Because his verdict was *nei ding*, meaning that it was decided at the higher level but not publicly announced, I had no idea that I was under supervision the whole time I was working at the hospital. This explained why I was always being sent down to the countryside and not allowed to attend certain meetings in the hospital. I was completely shocked, feeling angry and betrayed.

The rally against President Ding was scheduled, but because of the sexual nature of the matter, no one cared to be the speaker who had to denounce him in public. The committee appointed me to be the speaker.

"No," I said to them. "I'm not good at public speaking. I'll freeze up in front of so many people."

"You are a doctor and you know how to explain the matter. It will be much more convincing if you give a speech. Besides, you are a party member and you have the responsibility."

"You have to find someone else. I have never spoken in public before," I said.

For several days, they were unable to find anyone willing to deliver the speech, and I was afraid that they might force me to do it. It turned out that my worry was unnecessary. Dr. Chen had volunteered for the job. He wanted a chance to reform himself, but in reality he had hated President Ding ever since the Anti-Rightist movement and blamed Ding for having trapped him into a bad situation.

Just two weeks before the mass rally, President Ding, escorted by two Red Guards, had come in to see a doctor. He had liver disease. With his yellowish face and bloated stomach filled with excess fluid, he had to stand in line just like an average patient. First he sought out the doctors whom he had listed as "good" in his secret file. But the "good" doctors refused to examine him. They didn't want to see a counter-revolutionary patient. Even though he treated me badly when he was in power, I felt sorry for him, and gave him a three-day sick leave, so he could take a break from the hard manual labor. He was very grateful, but the two Red Guards became very angry. They tore the sick leave to pieces and said that I was sympathizing with a counter-revolutionary. But I told them that I was practicing the "revolutionary humanitarianism" that Chairman Mao advocated, and they couldn't argue with that.

The rally was held in the canteen where Ding used to hold meetings. The well-fed cooks were often used as thugs during the rallies. Before the meeting started, people were chatting and smoking. The smoke hung heavily over the meeting hall. Many people had cultivated the habit of smoking to kill time during the long political meetings.

I sat there for almost an hour but the meeting hadn't gotten underway. I watched some people running around on stage moving tables and chairs, as if preparing props for a play. Someone was testing the loudspeakers, which emitted a very irritating, ear-piercing screech. Then I heard gentle taps into the microphone, which was covered by a piece of bright red silk. *"Wei, wei."* The person spoke into the microphone, and adjusted its angle. There was a row of tables and chairs where the representatives from the Hospital Revolution Committee including hospital leaders, army officers, and Red Guards were gradually taking seats.

"I declare the mass rally officially begun!" a Red Guard from the Red Coat Battle Regiment solemnly announced at the top of his lungs. The loudspeakers screeched again. The speaker tapped on it a few times. After that had failed to stop the screeching, he just ignored it, and let it run its course.

"Bring the counter-revolutionary Ding onto the stage!" the Red Guard shouted after delivering a long-winded opening speech. Everyone's eyes opened wide as the Red Guards escorted President Ding onto the stage.

When the time came for Dr. Chen to speak, he went out of his way to explain the case in great medical detail, even though there were children and high school students in the audience. Of course, that was nothing unusual during a mass rally, where I had heard worse things. People were listening with thrilled attention. After the shocking details were revealed, a loud buzz erupted throughout the meeting hall.

"Down with the counter-revolutionary Ding!" the angry crowd yelled.

"Leniency for those who confess. Severity for those who resist!"

President Ding was made to stand on the chair, and bend at a sharp angle with a heavy wooden board that bore his name hung from his neck by a thin wire that dug deeply into his flesh. As the session proceeded, the violence intensified.

"Take him down, and step a foot on him to make sure he will never get up for the rest of his life!" People shouted the popular slogan.

That was just what they did to him. They kicked the chair over. President Ding hit the floor with great force. He was prodded back onto the chair and then kicked off it repeatedly until he could no longer stand up. When they flattened him on the ground, "the masses" all stormed onto the stage, and not just one but hundreds of feet stomped heavily on President Ding's bloated stomach. I wasn't sure what they were implying when they said "step a foot on him." Did they mean to step with one person's foot or with one of everyone's? Was the phrase just a metaphor? All I knew was that it was painful for him to have one foot on his stomach, not to mention hundreds.

During the mass rally, the army officers stayed on the sidelines, and only when the violence escalated did they stand up and shout Mao's slogan: "Fight with words; not violence." However, the crowd was "burning with righteous indignation." Nobody could have stopped them. Besides, the army officers were instructed by high level authorities not to interfere with the civilian struggles. Ding had offended many people when he was in power.

The meeting lasted until eleven o'clock at night. After the Red Coat Regiment had done with President Ding, the Yan'an Battle Regiment dragged him away for another session.

Next morning, I was woken up by the blare of the loudspeaker. It started with static for a few seconds, and the song "The East Is Red" — a paean to the savior Chairman Mao — suddenly blasted out. Then a harsh, ear-piercing female voice, filled with intense fervor, declared that the daily broadcast had officially begun.

There were urgent knocks on the door.

"Dr. Li," President Ding's wife, a nurse, shouted. "Quick! Something's wrong with old Ding! I came home from my night shift this morning and he's not breathing."

I immediately went over. President Ding, black and blue, was already stiff. Big chunks of his hair were missing, along with many of his teeth. He had been beaten to death that night. The Red Guards had hauled the corpse back to his home, put it on the bed, and left.

The mass rallies during the Cultural Revolution known as "struggle sessions" were too common, and quite often people were "struggled to death." Without any apparent reason the frenzied young people hated Ding; many of them came from outside the hospital and didn't even know who he was. Then there were people who were mistreated by Ding when he was in power, and they took their revenge on him. There was a doctor who had been forced to the countryside to do manual labor when she was five months' pregnant. As a result, she lost her baby. "There are many peasant women pregnant for many months and still working in the fields," Ding said sarcastically to her. "Why are you so fragile?" She had resented him ever since and during the rallies, she settled the old score with him. I often heard people say that some leaders were no good and didn't really care about "the masses," so when the political movement came, thank Chairman Mao for that, the people could exact their revenge. The oppressed are just as cruel as their oppressors. What a vicious circle! Even though Ding had refused to give me a leave, had forbidden me to seek better treatment for my son Bingbing years ago, and had also black-listed me as a "class alien," I couldn't find it inside myself to get even with him. In fact, I pitied him after his downfall.

15

SEPARATION

ON A NIGHT IN early October 1968, I packed everything for Wende: toothbrush, extra clothes, some snacks, and Chairman Mao's Little Red Book. Just like he had speculated before, the officials above the regimental level in 201 Division were going to Beijing to see Chairman Mao. He was very excited. The weather was not very cold at the time, but I still packed a sweater for him just in case. Today, I still keep this moth-eaten sweater in a wooden box as a witness to history.

"Finally, I will see Chairman Mao," Wende said as he pinned Chairman Mao's badge on the left side of his uniform, together with the honorable badges he had been awarded during his military career.

On Sunday, Wende came home unexpectedly. There was a lost look on his face.

"I thought you went to Beijing to see Chairman Mao," I said.

"They told me to stay and take care of things at the camp," he said. "Something is not right."

"Don't be paranoid. It's not a big deal. There will be so many people there, you won't be able to see Chairman Mao anyway. You can see him in movies and newspapers all the time," I said, trying to console him.

"Something is wrong," Wende kept saying. "Remember that the leaders in the political department once said that we had people among us who had worked for the Japanese before liberation? I think they were implying that I was the one. Now it is much more obvious than before. Otherwise, why would they suddenly cancel my trip for no reason?"

Wende was a man of few words and his history was a mystery to me. That was the first time he told me about his past in any detail.

"My father died when he was only forty," Wende told me. "When I was twelve I had to quit school and work in a small tailor shop in Tianjin to support my family. Then, later, my elementary schoolteacher became an officer in the police station during the Japanese occupation. When I was fourteen, he got me a job at the station. He was actually an underground Communist, and often instructed me to deliver messages to the Communist Party. When I was seventeen, he introduced me to the Communist Eighth Route Army. I told the army everything about my history, and they acknowledged that I was an underground Communist. In fact they placed six large seals onto my personal file as proof that the Communist Party was fully aware of the fact."

"Then don't worry about it. The party knows your history. You are an underground Communist. Why would they want to change the story?" I asked.

My effort to calm him down didn't work. When there was something on his mind, he would think about it over and over. He just couldn't ignore it.

The constant blare of the loudspeaker was driving me crazy. At the end of the day, the Communist song, "The Internationale," was played: "Rise, you poor hungry slaves. Rise, you suffering people of the world . . . the Internationale will fulfill." The loudspeaker broadcast finally came to an end after the song. The night became tranquil. Wende tossed around restlessly in the bed and sighed constantly.

I woke up in the middle of night and found him perched up in the bed with his coat around his shoulders. I didn't know how long he had been sitting like that.

"I have been thinking," he said. That was usually the way he opened the conversation. "If it comes to the worst, my elementary teacher can always testify for me. He knows all my history."

We analyzed everything all over again until we both were mentally and physically exhausted, but things still seemed unsettled.

While his colleagues were in Beijing for several days, Wende paced up and down the room with his hands behind his back, just like a caged animal. During that time, he was unable to eat or sleep, and developed many blisters on his lips from anxiety.

When the group came back from Beijing, one of Wende's comrades showed up with a photo. "Look, who is this?" he asked us.

I took the photo and examined it for a while. "Who's the fat old lady beside you?" I asked.

The comrade laughed but suddenly stopped and said solemnly, "That's not a fat old lady. It's our great leader, Chairman Mao!"

"Chairman Mao looks very healthy," Wende said, cutting in to relieve the awkwardness.

After the comrade left, Wende was very upset with me. "How could you say things so casually? Are you afraid that they won't be able to find fault with us?"

"It's just a mistake. He looked like a fat old lady in the picture. I didn't do it on purpose."

In the winter of 1968, the 201 Division of the 67 Army was ordered to relocate. Wende had started preparing for the big move weeks earlier. He didn't want to leave it for the last minute. Before we moved out of the military camp, Luping contracted hepatitis A. He had been sharing bones with his dog. He was just three years old. He liked to wear overall jeans with two pockets on the chest where he always stored some bones, which he and his dog took turns chewing on. He stayed in the 201 Division hospital for a couple of weeks before returning home. A nurse from the hospital came to spray our home with disinfectant.

"Don't eat his leftovers," I said to the old nanny. "I don't want you to catch the disease."

"There's no problem, why waste perfectly good food?" the old nanny said. She didn't listen to me.

From then on, Luping was not allowed to share bones with the dog or to feed it. At mealtime, he would stuff his mouth full of food and then go outside to feed his dog. A week later, when he went out to feed his dog some bones after supper, he saw his dog had been hanged on a tree with its eyes rolling back into its head. His cousin, who came from the countryside for a visit, was beating it with a stick.

Everyone in the camp had their share of the meat. Luping's cousin brought me one piece to the hospital but didn't tell me what kind of meat it was. I assumed it was pork because it tasted no different. After they told me it was Luping's pet, I became violently sick, throwing it all up in my office. I remembered that every time I came home, the dog would eagerly come running up from far away to greet me.

The night before the trip we were packing. We didn't have a lot of furniture, the major pieces consisting of only six huge wooden boxes. We had eight in total and two of them were at my apartment at the hospital. Even today, after some forty years, I still find it hard to part with those family treasures. Like the old saying goes: even a rundown home is worth a fortune. Since our family moved frequently, Wende became a very skilled packer. He packed everything very carefully. He wrapped the major pieces with straw mattresses, then tied them up very tightly with straw ropes. Smaller items were wrapped in old newspapers. In those days we had to be very cautious to make sure that Chairman Mao's photo was not in the newspaper that we used for wrapping; otherwise it would be a serious crime. The whole apartment was in chaos. Dust, straw, paper, and garbage were littered everywhere. Things that could never be found anywhere had surprisingly resurfaced. Cooking utensils and the wash basin were left to pack until the next morning. The children were all really excited about the trip.

At first Wende was told to go to Xuzhou, Jiangsu Province. But now he was instructed to go to a small village called Ceshan, Linyi County, in the south of Shandong Province, about one hundred miles away.

"Why is there a change of plan?" I asked.

"They said that while we were preparing, the Voice of America had already learned detailed information about the move," Wende said. Later, rumor had it that Wang Xiaoyu, the commander of Jinan Military District, was rebelling and it was his order to disperse the armies to different places in the name of exercises.

"How long will you be staying there?" I asked.

"I don't know. You have to keep working in the hospital. The children will come with me for now. If we stay there permanently, we'll just have to manage to get you transferred over there somehow," Wende said.

Early the next morning, I was woken up by the loud rumble of an engine. Someone was trying to start the truck in the cold morning. The truck heaved a heavy sigh and then there was a moment of silence. I knew that the person would try to get the vehicle started again. The sound of cranking the engine continued until it roared hysterically. Before long, the truck was running smoothly, its engine humming steadily. Truck after truck all started to warm up and hum continuously.

The windows were vibrating gently from the noise. It was still dark outside. We were all busy packing belongings the night before and didn't even have time to be sentimental. Now I was suddenly hit by the sad feeling of separation.

We loaded all of our belongings onto one big "liberation" truck. We had arranged that Luping, Yanping, and the babysitter would sit inside with the driver, while Wende and Xianping sat outside with the furniture. The truck roared several times before it finally set out from the military camp in Jiaonan, the fleet of trucks extending several miles. It was extremely cold so I gave Xianping a pair of woolen pants but he refused to wear them, instead just wearing an army overcoat. After the twelve-hour ride in the wintry conditions, he later developed arthritis in his knees.

Three weeks later, I received a long letter from Wende who described the situation there in detail:

> *Dear Qunying,*
> *How are you? We are all fine.*
>
> *We arrived at Ceshan in the evening. The water pipes were frozen solid so we had to melt snow for water. Many families had their castiron pots destroyed this way, because the cold snow on top and heat on the bottom would cause them to crack.*
>
> *Two days after we arrived there was a freezing rain. Icicles dangled from trees, and streets were coated with a sheet of ice that made them extremely slippery. Some soldiers suffered concussions after falling into the icy ditches.*
>
> *The babysitter took Yanping and Luping out to see an opera that was performed by the local Red Guard. The modern revolutionary model Beijing opera was Seizing the Tiger Mountain by Strategy. The old babysitter lost her footing several times on the way to the theater and back, either falling forward or backward. The old nanny's bound feet were too small to balance her even on normal ground, not to mention ice. The kids were all laughing at her.*
>
> *She also took Luping to see the Red Guard parade one day. She was trying to protect Luping from the firecrackers but she*

herself got hit by one, right on the nose. It bled heavily and she was really embarrassed by it. The old babysitter is very trustworthy. I gave her the money for all of the living expenses. Every time she goes to the market to buy groceries, she will tell Xianping to write it down and keep a record.

That's all for now. Revolutionary salutations!

Wende
January 1969

★

The 1969 Chinese New Year had arrived and I was all by myself. I had to work on New Year's Eve. I felt very sad. My family was hundreds of miles away and I missed them so much. At night, I heard the sporadic sound of firecrackers and the shouts of children. I didn't eat anything on New Year's Eve. In the morning, a nurse brought me some dumplings.

At first, I thought our family's separation was just temporary, since the hospital had promised to transfer me to Wende's location, but the days turned into months, and months turned into years. I had written several letters to Wende but never received any replies from him. I couldn't get a leave to go to see him and the kids. It reminded me of the situation during the Three-Anti's when our letters were cut off. It wasn't until much later that I found out that Wende was under investigation.

In the summer of 1969, as I was sleeping in my apartment, someone threw a letter in through the back window. The letter was unsigned. Apparently it was from Wende's old comrade Shouyi who had come back to visit his wife and children. He informed me about Wende's situation by scribbling a note and tossing it in through the window, because he was afraid of direct contact. The note, jam-packed with grammar and spelling mistakes, was hardly readable because he couldn't write well. I managed to understand.

Wende wants me to tell you everything is all right. In spring he was instructed to go to a military farm beside the Hongze Lake, Jiangsu Province, to join a study group. The farm is about two hundred miles from home. He has not come back since then. It's concerning his history problem. He trusts the party will clear the matter eventually.

I asked Shouyi to bring some photos of my kids next time. I missed them very much. Shouyi was one of the officials in charge of the "study group." He didn't think the way they were treating Wende was fair, but there was nothing he could do about it. He went back and told Wende about my request. Two months later, upon receiving a photo, I was so upset that I tore the picture into pieces. I thought that the children's picture would comfort me, but it was just the opposite. I became even more worried. Yanping and Luping both looked very unhappy. I could pretty much tell that the life there was miserable just from one look at the photo.

Later, I learned that throughout the course of being in the study group, Wende returned only once to visit the children. During that short visit, he took Yanping and Luping to town to have a quick picture taken. It wasn't easy to find a photo shop in the countryside. The military camp was eight miles away from town, so he had to carry the children by bike, one at a time because he was unable to carry both of them together. He would ride with Yanping for one mile, drop her off, come back to get Luping, and repeat the whole laborious process many times. The road was in terrible condition. During the rainy days earlier, the vehicles had made deep ruts in the muddy road. When dry, the road became very bumpy to ride on. He had to be very careful because on both sides of the road were deep reed marshes. I could imagine that Wende wasn't in a good mood, which would also explain why the children all looked so sad in the photo.

Just recently, I looked again at our old family photo album. I thought there was a negative of this photo but I couldn't find it anywhere. The photo would really help to explain this part of our history. This was the time when our family was split into three parts, hundreds of miles from each other for close to two years. It wasn't until much later that I learned the details about their lives during my two-year absence from Wende and Xianping.

When they first got to Linyi, the army camp was in a huge disarray, littered everywhere with damaged military supplies. It was apparent that a fierce fight had taken place at an auditorium not long before. Blood stained the walls and all the windows were broken. The doors were blocked by sandbags for protection. On the roof, there were bullet holes of different sizes. The 68 Army that changed posts with the 67 Army also belonged to the Jinan Military District. The 68 Army had interfered with the struggles of the local Red Guard rival factions. The local Red Guard Rebels had used weapons they had seized from the 68 Army to attack the heavily fortified auditorium. There were deaths and injuries on both sides.

There was a Red Guard Rebel organization, called Maling Mountain Guerrillas, who threatened to seize the soldiers' weapons. The children in the camp were told not to play outside of the residential compound. The sirens often sounded at midnight.

A new soldier from Sichuan was nearsighted, and always nervous when he was on sentry duty at night to guard the residential compound. One night he heard something and opened fire. He ended up killing a villager's dog. As if faced with a formidable foe, the siren went off and the whole army was put on high alert. Scared to patrol at night, the soldier often sneaked over to Wende's apartment to play with the children.

The housewives and children all went to see a pig at the army's farm. The pig had been severely deformed with a knife by a soldier from the 68 Army previously stationed there, possibly because of the bitter hatred that existed between the different factions among the armies. The women and children watched the pig with horror, unable to even determine what the animal was.

Chinese New Year came not long after Wende and the children settled down in Linyi. They spent the 1969 Spring Festival in the cold and cheerless atmosphere without me. Limited quantities of pig head and feet, meat and eggs were allotted. No one was allowed to buy more. The mood also wasn't so festive because the old traditions and customs, such as setting off firecrackers and wearing new clothes, were discouraged. All the children in the residential compound wore old army uniforms. The only difference between the New Year and any ordinary day was that people were having better meals during the holiday.

Shortly after the New Year, Wende was assigned the job of managing the military farm at Tancheng County over eighty miles away. Military farming was an old tradition that kept the army self-sufficient. Since he was very anxious to start work and there wasn't a vehicle available at the time to get him there, he got up at the crack of dawn and walked the entire day on an unfamiliar winding country road to the farm. He lost his way a couple of times and almost reached the border of Jiangsu Province. Several huge blisters covered his feet from the long march. He often stayed at the farm for days, then walked all the way back. That was how devoted he was to his work.

He didn't work there for long, and in the spring he was ordered to go to a military farm beside the Hongze Lake in Jiangsu Province to join a study group — just as his old comrade Shouyi described in a short note. The so-called study group was, of course, just another concentration camp — this one for the military officials from 67 and 68 Armies who had political problems. These officers were forced to do backbreaking labor, such as transplanting rice seedlings, bending the whole day in water that was infested with all kinds of parasites. All through the night, they had to write confessions.

There was no freedom in the camp, and they were closely watched at all times by armed soldiers.

Afraid that I would worry, Wende pleaded with Shouyi not to tell me about his real situation. So that explained why in his note Shouyi had said everything was fine. But instinct told me it was far from that. Even today, I still don't know exactly what happened at the study group, because it was too painful for Wende to talk about.

This was the darkest time for our family. During the beginning of the Cultural Revolution, my family was almost untouchable. Then came the Cleanse the Class Ranks campaign (1968–1970), the peak of the Cultural Revolution, aimed to uncover the political dissidents: landlords, rich peasants, counter-revolutionaries, bad elements who hadn't been reformed; rightists who had slipped through the nets; traitors, spies, and unrepentant capitalist roaders. This campaign to purify the class ranks was the most brutal phase of the Cultural Revolution. The broadness of people purged, the brutality due to the hatred between the different factions, and the death toll exceeded that of the beginning phases of the Cultural Revolution — including the red terror of the young Red Guard, the armed conflicts among the Rebels, and possibly all previous political campaigns. According to one estimate, during the Cleanse the Class Ranks campaign alone, over a half million people were killed and thirty million were denounced, humiliated, and tortured. If the Red Guard rampage and Rebel armed conflicts were "spontaneous" mass movements, then Cleanse the Class Ranks was directly overseen by Mao himself; it was a systematical witch hunt of millions of real or imagined dissidents. The scope of persecution expanded so broadly that no one, including Rebels, felt safe anymore, and everyone was trying to protect themselves, even by means of telling lies or selling out others. Many officials with "bad class origin" — namely landlords or those with capitalist family backgrounds and those who were arrested during either the Japanese occupation or the Nationalist regime — were now suspected of being traitors or spies. All were interrogated, tortured, killed, or driven to suicide.

During the Cleanse the Class Ranks, Kang Sheng emerged as a notorious security chief. He was compared to Dzerzhinsky, the founder of the Cheka — the Bolshevik secret police and the predecessor of the KGB — known for his ruthless elimination of counter-revolutionaries during the Lenin era. Back in 1933, Kang was sent to Moscow where he studied Soviet security and intelligence techniques. In 1942, Mao and Kang started the Yan'an Rectification campaign which Kang turned into a witch hunt for "Nationalist spies," and a physical and psychological persecution of dissidents. He became an adviser to the Cultural Revolution Group, which was formed in May 1966 and consisted of the other four radicals Jiang Qing, Chen Boda, Yao Wenyuan, and Zhang Chunqiao. In 1968, Kang became the chief of the secret police, and took control of the Central Investigation Department.

He launched a campaign against members of the former Inner Mongolian People's Party, which had been dismissed in the mid thirties and absorbed by the Communist Party in the late forties. One estimate shows that over 87,000 people were disabled by torture during the interrogation and the death toll reached over 16,000 in this deadly witch hunt. In another case, without any grounds, Kang accused the secretary of Yunnan Provincial Party Committee of being a Nationalist spy, and ordered his arrest and an immediate hunt for his spy network. Over a million people were implicated, 17,000 were beaten to death or driven to suicide, and 60,000 were disabled by torture. Kang was directly involved in the purges of Liu Shaoqi, Deng Xiaoping, Peng Dehuai, and many other high-ranking leaders.

Liu Shaoqi was attacked during the early stages of the Cultural Revolution as a revisionist with the charges escalating into treason and "the No. 1 capitalist roader" in 1967. He and his wife were publicly humiliated during the Red Guard mass rallies. In October 1968, the Central Committee passed a resolution to expel him from the party. He died mysteriously the following year while in captivity, with speculations ranging from medical neglect all the way to murder. Deng Xiaoping, the No. 2 capitalist roader, was also purged, but somehow managed to ride the political roller coaster for the next decade until his glorious comeback in 1977. Peng Dehuai, the only person who stood up to Mao during the Great Leap Forward, was crippled by the Red Guard. Denied medical treatment, he died in 1974.With the fall of the top leaders, Kang Sheng quickly rose to the number-four figure just behind Mao, Lin, and Zhou. He became the most feared "butcher" in the internal power struggle of the Communist Party.

By that time, the "capitalist roaders" Liu Shaoqi, Deng Xiaoping, and their followers had been brought down with the help of the young Red Guard. At the end of 1968, after the young troublemakers finished their historical mission, Mao, with no further need for them, issued an order to send young people in flocks to the remote corners of the country. The enormous numbers of frantic young people in the cities had become a threat to political stability. Young people across the nation immediately followed Mao's order and headed out into the isolated countryside where, for years, they were subjected to poor and backward conditions. There were more than 16 million of them in total. Many of them were full of enthusiasm and volunteered to go to the countryside, while some were forced by the government to leave their homes.

On many occasions I was approached by parents who didn't want their children to go to the countryside. I was asked to fake medical records to show that their children had illnesses that could help them avoid the hardship. In most cases, I couldn't find any health problems with the kids although their parents were often sick from worry. It wasn't until years after the Cultural Revolution ended that many of these young people received permission to return home to their families in the cities, at which point they became bitterly disillusioned and felt that many years of their valuable lives had been cheated from them.

In March 1969, border clashes broke out between Soviet and Chinese troops over Zhenbao Island, a place less than one square kilometer in the Ussuri River. There were casualties on both sides. After the conflicts, there were about one and a half million troops deployed along the border. It was a part of the Cold War age. Meanwhile, Chairman Mao ordered the whole country to prepare for imminent war. Extensive networks of air-raid tunnels were swiftly constructed under cities and important military bases, and factories were moved underground. According to the older residents in Jinan, a city well known for its beautiful springs, the concrete underground construction had blocked the fountainheads, causing the springs to dry up.

In Wende's military camp, each household was instructed to dig a hole in its yard spacious enough to hide the whole family and to store a six-month supply of food in case of nuclear war. Each family received a manual on what to do if a nuclear bomb struck. There were drills too. Every time they heard the wail of the siren, the children and the babysitter would drop whatever they were doing, sometimes in the middle of supper, rush into the shelter, and stay put until further notice was given. Shouyi and some other officers were sent by the army to advise the civilians on how to build bomb shelters. Of course, years went by and the nuclear war people had diligently prepared for never came. I heard that some people utilized the bomb shelters as personal storage spaces, sometimes secretly hiding Four Olds in them. In the major cities, many of these tunnels are used as underground markets today.

For about three months after Wende and the children arrived in Linyi, Xianping couldn't find a school. It usually took some time for the military officers to arrange their children's schooling with the local government. Xianping often walked through the camp to salvage some damaged military supplies, like knives, water bottles, and leather bags. He was keen on mountain climbing, swimming, and wrestling with the new recruits at the army base. He was thirsty for knowledge, but there were few books available in those days except Chairman Mao's works. Before leaving for the study group, Wende had given Xianping two books: one was called *Political Economy* written by a Russian author, and the other one titled *Military Topography*.

In the springtime, Xianping went to the Linyi Tenth High School several miles away. He had to bring his own lunch, a couple of cold buns. At lunch time, Xianping would go outside the school to eat because he didn't want his classmates, mostly poor country kids, to see him eating. Since buns were considered a luxury, he didn't want give the poor children a feeling of inequality.

Because the kids of Xianping's age rarely went to school and often caused trouble, in the fall 1969, the residents' committee in the compound rounded them all up and sent them to the 201 division's military farm at Tancheng County to do manual labor. This was the farm where Wende had previously worked. When Xianping got there, he saw his father's bed and some of his belongings still there. This told Xianping that Wende had left for the study group in a hurry. The children all lived with soldiers in the damp adobes. The work involved harvesting crops by cutting soybean plants with a sickle, and threshing rice with a simple threshing machine that had a cylinder with spikes on it. One kid would peddle to make the machine turn while two kids would feed plants into it. At mealtime, everyone ate squatting down; there were no tables or chairs to sit on. Even though it was a hard life, the kids seemed to like the farm work better than going to school. During that time, Xianping became interested in drawing, always having a how-to-draw book with him. He didn't have a teacher though so he didn't get too far with it.

In spring, Yanping went to a school in Ceshan village, a couple of miles away. The classroom was set up in an adobe house with the desks also made of a mixture of mud and straw. According to her, even if you entered the classroom on a sunny day, it would take a long time for your eyes to adjust to the darkness before you could see anything. In summer, she often went out at night with the wives in the residential compound to dig for cicadas under the trees. The cicada is a large-sized insect that lives underground as larva for up to seventeen years before it comes to the surface of the earth. At the age of nine, Yanping was fascinated by these creatures. She would put them on the window screen and watch them shed their shells and turn into adults, each with a pair of transparent, veined wings. The abandoned shells of cicadas are often found still clinging onto the bark of trees, and are commonly used as an ingredient in Chinese medicine to treat colds, sore throat, measles, spasms, eye disorders, and many other illnesses. The locals had the habit of eating the fried larva. Yanping also took up the hobby of planting wild flowers around the front of the door and was very serious about it.

Luping often went to the stable in the army camp to see the military horses, or to the pigsty to watch the piglets being fed. The old babysitter with her bound feet could hardly keep up with him. If she couldn't find him, she would go to check out the deep well in the yard, worried that the boy might have accidentally fallen into it because he frequently played near the site. Often he would play on the hill behind the residential compound with some kids his age. He dug many sizable holes in the ground and then put water or other traps into them before covering them up perfectly. He even took off his shoes to gently place footprints over the areas to camouflage them, then waited for someone to step on them. Sometimes he would tie a piece of wood on a string, bury it underground, and then pull the string when someone passed by to give them a good scare. He learned these tricks in a propaganda movie called *Mine War*, one of only a few movies showing in those years. Luping maintained this hobby for many years.

Even though the nanny was kind and trustworthy, the old country woman was not a neat and tidy person. That was the cause of Luping suffering with a bout of worms. Roundworm disease among children was very common those days due to poor sanitation. The nanny was not a good cook by any means. They usually dined on a stir-fry of cabbage or turnips with steamed buns or rice while sitting on four small chairs in front of a very low table. Nevertheless, our family owed a great deal to her for helping out during those years when Wende and I were away from home. In fact, our children were the only ones in the residential compound without both parents at home but just an old nanny. She was a hard worker and during that time she had to stay in the hospital for a week because of the severe arthritis in her hands that was so painful that she couldn't even sleep at night.

16

THE INNERMOST SOUL

ON THE VERY FIRST DAY of 1970, when I went to the hospital canteen, I accidentally dropped and broke my china bowl. "You're going to lose your job," a colleague of mine joked. The bowl was a symbol of one's livelihood. Only a few short months later, the joke became a reality.

Just a few months later, in April, I was summoned to see the hospital revolution committee. When I went into the office, I saw four serious-looking people in the office: the head of the committee, two Red Guards, and an army officer. The atmosphere sent sweat down my spine.

"The ambulance driver has exposed you. A patient died because of your negligence," a Red Guard said.

"What are you talking about?" I said.

"The driver said you sat in the driver's cab of the ambulance while the patient was suffering at the back. You're responsible for the boy's death. As a doctor, how could you leave the patient alone, unattended?"

"It's not true. I was with the patient all the time. I can't believe he would say something like that," I told them.

Two days before, I had gone in an ambulance to see a patient who lived in a village about fifty miles away. When we finally reached the village, it was too late. The boy was extremely ill with pneumonia from measles complications. His lips had already turned dark. It would take at least an hour to get back to the hospital. I gave him a cardiac stimulant in the ambulance. I was in the back of the ambulance with the patient the whole time. In fact, my fingers were on the boy's pulse the whole way. As we got closer to the hospital, the boy's pulse died away. I did everything I could to save him but his pulse stopped before we reached the hospital. I knew how sad the mother would be, because my second son, Bingbing, also died from measles complications.

"The boy had already died. The mother must feel very sad. Let's not charge them the ambulance fee or the fee for making a house call," I said to the ambulance driver.

"Fine, you sign the paper. I'm not responsible for this," he said.

So I signed the documents. Carrying the dead boy in her arms, the mother walked all the way home.

How could the driver accuse me of negligence? I couldn't think of any explanation. I had never offended him in any way. In fact, before Wende's problem surfaced, I had gone with this driver on emergencies many times in the past. We had a very good relationship. My kids used to like him and often took rides with him in the ambulance.

I told the committee my side of the story. They approached the family to investigate the matter. The boy's mother told them the truth. "Yes, the doctor was with my child all the time," she said to them. I didn't know what would happen if the family decided to testify against me for some reason. Right now, I couldn't afford to give the hospital any excuse to hold something against me. However, as the saying goes, "Anything that can go wrong will go wrong." That was definitely true in my case.

While Wende was ordered to write a confession in the so-called study group, the hospital started putting pressure on me. They put up posters to criticize me, and called me the "counter-revolutionary's wife," "Nationalist Spy," or "black person of dubious background," a phase which indicated my past was in question. The people from the hospital revolution committee often furnished information about me to Wende's army, and, in turn, the army informed the hospital about Wende's situation. "Your father is a traitor and a counter-revolutionary. Your mother is a spy, and you're a son of bitch," Xianping's classmates said to him in school.

I had no idea what was happening to Wende in the study group. Later on, I learned from Xianping that during a short visit, Wende had taken him to town, bought him a pair of leather shoes, and, on the way, said, "Your mother's problem is very serious. We can't live with her anymore."

Those words made a very deep impression on my fifteen-year-old son, although he couldn't figure out exactly what Wende really meant. What had they been telling Wende about me? Later it became clear to me what a state of confusion and pressure Wende must have been under, for him to have doubted me. There was no question that he was broken psychologically, if not physically.

A few days later, I was called into the office again. The same people who had interrogated me earlier were present. This time they asked me many questions about my personal history.

"Everyone has a home — why don't you have one?" a Red Guard questioned.

"It's not my fault I don't have a family. My mother died when I was very young and my father went missing," I said.

"Missing? What happened?"

"He ran away when the Japanese were rounding people up as slaves."

"That sounds very suspicious to me. What about your relatives?"

"I lost all contact with my hometown when the troop left Chifeng."

"Were you a Nationalist before you joined the Eighth Route Army?" another Red Guard asked. "Are you a spy?"

"No, I'm not."

"What's your class origin?" the head of the committee asked.

"The urban poor."

"We heard that you were from a rich capitalist family who exploited people before liberation. You have to confess everything."

"There's nothing to confess. I was from a poor family. We didn't exploit anyone," I said.

The hospital revolutionary committee was not convinced. They assumed that if my husband had problems then I might have problems too. So they sent a four-person investigation group to my hometown, Chifeng, to gather some information about me. One of the investigators was a doctor from the X-ray Department. Another was a copy clerk. After two weeks of investigation and sightseeing in the city, they returned, deeply impressed by the city.

"Say, Chifeng is a nice place!" an investigator said to me.

After the investigators came back, I was called into the office again. "You are not cooperating with our investigation. Because of that we had to waste money and travel a long way to your hometown to collect information. And now we have enough evidence against you. We want to give you a last chance to come clean," the head of the committee said.

"I have already told you everything," I said. "And what evidence do you have?"

"We have found a photo. And it can explain everything," he said.

It was an old picture of my mother and me posing with my cousin.

"Where did you get it?" I asked.

"From your relatives."

"I didn't even know I still have relatives there," I said.

"Judging by the picture, you don't look like you were from a poor family. Look, you and your mother were wearing sliver bracelets, silk robes, and leather shoes," a Red Guard said.

"The urban poor would rather go hungry, but dress decently," I told him. "Can I keep the picture?"

"No, you can't have it. It's evidence now."

The conclusion of the investigation was that my confession was "basically true." After the investigation, the picture was returned to me. They didn't give the name of the relative who provided the photo. They told me that the photo was taken out of a frame that was mounted on the wall. I suspected that this relative could be my long-lost cousin in the photo. All of my belongings, including my childhood pictures, had been lost during the escape from Chifeng in 1946, when the Nationalists raided our ammunition factory. Thanks to the investigators, at least one childhood photo was recovered. That was the only photograph ever preserved of my mother. It brought back many memories for me.

As I studied the group portrait, I was overwhelmed by the grave facial expressions and the rigid positions in which the subjects were arranged. The wrinkled, dark appearance of the photo intensified the grim atmosphere. I couldn't remember which year it was taken. It might have been taken the year before my mother died. I assumed that it was indeed a special occasion since photo studios during that time were exceedingly rare.

Dr. Chen was considered to be the best surgeon in the city and he was very proud of that fact. His class origin aggravated him when he had to fill out a registration form during the Cleanse the Class Ranks. Every time there was a political movement, people had to fill out forms to indicate their family background and their "political behavior" in the movement. Concerned about his family history, he couldn't sleep or eat for days. He asked me for my advice on how he should fill out the question about his class background.

"Big Sister," he said. "How should I fill this out? Should I put down capitalist?"

"Capitalist refers to the people who had assets before liberation. How could you be a capitalist at your age?" I said.

"My grandfather was a capitalist before liberation. After liberation they converted his private business to national ownership and my father became a clerk. I had nothing to do with capitalism. If I am a capitalist, my children and my grandchildren would be capitalists too. You are a party member, and you are a big sister to me. What do you think I should do?"

"The Communists are supposed to eliminate classes eventually, not to expand them. I'll mention your case to Commissar Feng when I have a chance to see him and find out what his opinion is. I'll put in a few good words for you. For the time being, don't worry too much about it," I said to him. He was very grateful to me. There wasn't anybody else willing to talk to him at all.

While Dr. Chen was worrying about his family history, Commissar Feng developed kidney disease that might require surgery. Dr. Chen was the only one qualified for the job. It was a perfect time for me to talk to Commissar Feng about Dr. Chen's class origin problem. But things didn't go as I had expected. Dr. Chen examined the commissar and informed him that he needed surgery to have one of his kidneys removed.

"Those surgeons, they are so eager to cut you up!" the commissar said sarcastically.

Commissar Feng didn't really trust Dr. Chen's diagnosis, or maybe he didn't trust Dr. Chen himself. Whatever the reason, he hurried off to Shanghai for a second opinion. The conclusion was the same. Commissar Feng figured that if he underwent the operation in Shanghai, no one would lavish any attention on him since he was no one there. On the other hand, he would be treated like a king here in Jiaonan County. So he came back and wanted Dr. Chen to operate on him. Dr. Chen, who had been subjected to all kinds of indignities, still possessed his professional pride. He felt humiliated and refused to perform the surgery for the commissar. "I'm not qualified. Find someone else," he said.

Commissar Feng was outraged. "That arrogant stinky intellectual. This is the people's hospital. If he doesn't serve the proletariat, who else does he serve? The bourgeoisie?" he said.

The commissar didn't trust anyone else in the hospital. In the end, he relied upon his connections and arranged for a surgeon from Shanghai to come and perform the operation in Jiaonan. In that way, he had the best surgeon from a big city and all the convenience they could provide in a small community. Shortly afterward, Dr. Chen, escorted by Red Guards armed with big sticks, was sent down to the countryside again to reform through hard labor. Every time he sneaked back to visit his family, he would be beaten up and sent away again.

In June, Commissar Feng called me to his ward and wanted to have a chat with me. He occupied the entire east wing of the hospital ward, guarded by armed soldiers so that no one could get closer than fifty meters without permission. Since only he and his female secretary occupied the wing, the ward was very quiet. The rest of the ward was crammed full, many patients having no choice but to lie on beds in the hallway. Rumor had it that Commissar Feng had gotten his pretty female secretary pregnant and forced her to marry his male secretary to hide the fact. Despite the rumors about him, people still had great respect for Commissar Feng.

"How are you feeling, Commissar?" I asked.

"Much better," the commissar said. "The surgeon came from Shanghai. He is one of the best in the country."

"Why did you need to get a surgeon from Shanghai? We have a good surgeon right here."

"Oh, you mean Dr. Chen. He's a rightist, an intellectual snob. I'd rather die than let a counter-revolutionary operate on me." The commissar sat up in the bed.

"Comrade Qunying, I couldn't be more sympathetic about your situation," Commissar Feng said. "I know you don't deserve this, but I warned you in the past about Han Wende. I knew his history. There's not much I can do for you now. But if you draw a clear line between your husband and yourself by divorcing him, I can put in some good words for you with the hospital revolution committee to let you hold on to your job. Otherwise, you will have no other option but to leave for the countryside with him to reform through hard labor."

"Why would I divorce him when we have a good relationship? Besides, we have three children."

"That's exactly the point. Your husband is now a historical counter-revolutionary. He shouldn't drag you and your children into this mess."

"I can't desert my husband when he needs me the most."

"You're stubborn as usual. Haven't changed over the years. I only tell you this for old times' sake. If you change your mind, let me know, so I can talk to the committee, but the time is limited."

The people from the hospital and 201 Division all tried to convince me to divorce Wende, but they failed. In July of 1970, I was expelled from the hospital. I packed my suitcase and left to reunite with my family. I hadn't seen Wende and the kids for almost two years. A doctor and one of the former hospital officials who were being "reformed through hard labor" were assigned to carry my belongings — two big wooden boxes — to the bus station. There was no train in Jiaonan so I had to take a bus to Jiaoxian then take a train from there. At the time, the army had moved to Changluo County where a leprosy hospital was located on the top of a mountain not far from the army camp. All of the leprosy patients from the entire province were sent there for treatment. People were afraid to go anywhere near the place and always held their breath when passing the hospital, believing that the horrifying disease could be transmitted by air. At the time, leprosy was the most feared of all infectious diseases because it caused deformity, including skin lesions, nerve damage, and, in serious cases, loss of patients' fingers and toes. The disease is still not under control in some countries today.

Wende's friend Shouyi had secretly informed my family about my situation and my departure from the Jiaonan Hospital, but he didn't know the exact date, time, and the train number of my arrival in Changluo. So Xianping went to the train station by bike a couple of times each day to meet me. Occasionally he took five-year-old Luping with him. Luping would sit on the front of the bike with both of his hands on the handlebars. They had been disappointed many times when I failed to show up. Often they stopped at the railway crossing and looked into the fast-passing trains in hopes of spotting me inside.

On the train, I imagined the scene of when we met and how excited everyone would be. A few hours later, I finally arrived at the Changluo railway station with only a carry-on; the rest of my possessions were shipped separately and would get there in the following days. I hadn't seen my son for close to two years and couldn't recognize him at all until all the passengers had all left the station. When there were just the two of us left, we looked at each other. Xianping, already fifteen, had changed dramatically over the two years. He had grown taller and his voice had become deeper. A light mustache on his upper lip made him look a bit awkward. He was a little withdrawn and didn't seem as happy to see me as I had imagined.

Laying eyes on Wende and the kids, I broke into tears. Luping and Yanping couldn't even recognize me after almost two years apart. Wende looked dark from the hard labor at the military farm. He had lost a significant amount of weight and his hair had turned gray. His uniform had been stripped of badges, giving him a bare, awkward appearance. By that time, he had already left the study group.

"You shouldn't have come. You should have stayed at the hospital. The children can stay with you. I can go to the countryside by myself. There's no point in dragging you and the children into this mess," Wende said to me.

"It's no big deal," I said to him. "Let's all go. At least we will be together."

I looked around the apartment. It was neater than I had imagined. At the corner of the apartment, I found a plaster statue of Chairman Mao with half of its face missing.

"What happened to the statue?" I asked.

"The people who lived here before us left it. We didn't touch it," the old nanny said. "The officials came to question me about it. 'Did Han Wende do that?' they asked me. 'No,' I told them. 'It was like that when we first moved in. You people got it all wrong,' I said. 'Wende is a good man.'" The old nanny was always loyal to the family.

Chairman Mao's portrait was sacred. Every household had at least one or two, which were usually posted on the most prominent spots on the wall. There were also plaster statues. It was said that the steel made in the backyard furnaces during the Great Leap Forward was all very low grade and good for nothing, so they used it to make Mao badges of different shapes and sizes, which became collectors' items many years later.

At the apartment, I also came across a letter written by Wende intended for me. It was his last will.

> Dear Qunying,
> When you read this letter, I have already gone.
> I have dedicated my heart and soul to the revolution for twenty-five years, and I have boundless love and gratitude for our great leader Chairman Mao and the party. They told me that the confession should come from my innermost soul. What else could I tell them other than that I had worked underground for the Communists before liberation? I had

revealed that part of my history many times in the past. The first time was when I joined the army in 1945. I had told the army everything about myself and there are six stamps on my personal file as proof that the party was fully aware of my history. The second time was during the Three-Anti's while I was on the battlefield in Korea in 1952. The third time was in 1955, during the Cleanup of Counter-Revolutionaries Movement. And now I'm forced to confess again during the Cultural Revolution.

During the Cleanse the Class Ranks, they announced me as a historical counter-revolutionary who hid in the People's Army. I was expelled from the army and the party. Everyone drew a clear line between them and me. The deep feelings I had shared with my old comrades and chiefs all disappeared at once. Everyone treated me like an enemy. I was ordered to leave the army within a specified period of time and return to my hometown to reform through hard labor. It was really a situation of "I cry to the heaven and there is no reply; I call to the earth and there is no answer."

I had no choice but to classify myself as a counter-revolutionary. In a party membership meeting, they stripped the badges off my uniforms and then wanted me to make a statement. I said that the Communist Party is composed of advanced elements. I'm a counter-revolutionary and deserved to be expelled from the army and the party.

I don't want to drag you and the children into this mess. It's not fair for you and the children to suffer because of my problem. I hope someday they will prove that I'm innocent.

Revolutionary Salutations!
Wende
July 1970

"You should never think like that," I said to him. "Think about our children! What are they going to do without you?"

When I questioned him closely, he admitted that if I had arrived a few days later, he would have committed suicide just like his superior, Liu Shugang, whom people referred to as "loving the soldiers like his own sons." Liu had been charged with countless crimes and labeled a spy, traitor, counter-revolutionary, and more. Before he was sent to a labor camp, he hanged himself with his belt in the bathroom. If a person took his own life, it proved that he really was guilty. Suicide in itself was a crime because it meant that the person had "alienated himself from the people." It meant he was "so guilty that even death would not expiate all his crimes." During the Cleanse the Class Ranks campaign, a huge number of innocent officials committed suicide because they couldn't bear the humiliation of falling from grace, and the constant physical and psychological torment. Every time I think about this campaign, the word suicide comes into my mind. Under the tremendous pressure, people would simply become full of despair.

"I told them I was an underground Communist and my schoolteacher could testify to it for me. He was a very important official in the government in Tianjin. The officials from 201 Division sent some investigators to Tianjin and found that my teacher had also been brought down at the time. He wasn't even able to prove himself innocent," Wende told me.

It turned out that Wende's schoolteacher also needed someone to testify for himself, and the only person who could have proved his innocence had died. For safety purposes, members of the underground Communists only had one-way contact with each other, which meant that each member was only permitted to communicate with one other person. Therefore, if one member fell into enemy hands, he wouldn't be able to expose the entire network.

"It's not the physical labor I'm afraid of," Wende said. "It's the torment of the mind I can't bear." He often described the Cultural Revolution as an event that had "touched people to their innermost souls." Besides the factor of the Cleanse the

Class Ranks campaign, personal revenge also played a role in Wende's persecution. He had offended several officials by refusing to participate in the embezzling scheme in the early fifties and they had resented him ever since. This campaign offered them an opportunity to finally get back at him.

The damage of the Cultural Revolution and its aftermath was unprecedented. Some compared it to the French Revolution in terms of the chaos, blood, and destruction. Nearly everyone had suffered, from the young people like my son Xianping, deprived of a decade of education, to the scholars persecuted for owning Western books; from peasants at the grassroots level to the top leaders like the state chairman Liu Shaoqi, the party's general secretary Deng Xiaoping, and many other high-ranking officials. Everyone was in a constant state of fear, anxiety, and paranoia. Victimizers one day turned into victims the next and vice versa. The full history, including the death toll of the Cultural Revolution is still far from known. Many people were "struggled" to death, murdered, driven to suicide, exiled, or went mysteriously missing. Some sources estimate the death toll as high as seven million, with a median of one million. However, the trauma people sustained cannot be measured by numbers.

The night our family left for the countryside, the old nanny couldn't stop crying, tears streaming down her wrinkled, pockmarked face. In fact, she had started crying three days earlier and wanted to leave with our family.

"What's the point of coming with us? We are going to the countryside to do manual labor. You might as well go back home," I said to her.

The old babysitter had become just like one of our family, so it wasn't easy to let her go. After all those years of my being too busy to be with my children, the nanny was more of a mother to them — especially during the time when our family was split into three parts, hundreds of miles from each other. Over the years, the old nanny had become attached to the children. She cared for them as if they were her own. I knew how heavy-hearted she felt. I couldn't imagine what would happen to her, but we were in the situation of "like a clay idol fording a river — hardly able to save itself." All I could do was to leave the sad old woman some things she could use. Wende also gave her fifty yuan before we left.

At the time, a neighbor needed a babysitter. He had trouble keeping anyone because his wife would only give the babysitter leftovers to eat. The neighbor asked me: "They all say that you have a bad temper yet your babysitter is so good to you. Why?"

I told him: "I treat her like a member of my family."

"I don't really want to work for him," the old babysitter said, wiping her tears, her whole face twisted with sorrow.

"Why don't you try it out for a few days. If they treat you well, you stay. If not, leave," I said.

In July of 1970, on a hot summer night, our family left the military camp and headed for the train station in the pouring rain. No one came to see us off. People were all afraid to have anything to do with us, avoiding us as if we had the plague. Xianping carried Luping on his back. Luping was sleeping and unaware of what was going on. I was carrying a thermos bottle — a very valuable family possession wrapped with a towel. Shortly after we walked out of the apartment, I fell and was badly hurt on the slippery muddy road, but I protected the thermos by lifting it in the air so it didn't break. Luckily there was nobody around at that late hour; otherwise I would have been really embarrassed by it. Knowing Wende, even if not for this incident, he probably would have preferred that we left in the middle of night so that nobody would see us. How humiliating it would have been if people had been watching us being kicked out of the army in broad daylight. On the street near the train station, there were some people wearing black raincoats, shining under the streetlights like ghosts.

We had to change to another train at Jinan station. There were several windows open for selling tickets, but I had no idea which line I should be in. There were many people inside the waiting hall. The air was heavy, almost suffocating. Signs listing train numbers and destinations hung over each waiting line. When a train was ready, a railway attendant would remove the sign and lead the passengers to the boarding entrance.

This time, however, there were too many passengers. When the loudspeaker announced that it was time to board the train, it caused chaos. All the passengers tried to squeeze their way to the front of the line.

"Don't push! Form a line!" the railway attendant yelled, but her voice was drowned out by the crowd. Suspecting that the situation would turn ugly, the attendant sneaked her way to the back of the line, secretly leading passengers to the boarding entrance. In that way, the end of the line became the front. This was a commonly used trick in cases where there were too many passengers. By the time people at the front of the line discovered that they had been fooled, it was already too late. With children, we couldn't fight the crowd.

It became a free-for-all with people shoving and cutting into the line. At that moment, everyone seemed to have lost any sense of self-esteem. I felt like an animal being herded into a pen. The crowd was a big wave, carrying us back and forth, left and right, with no control at all. The only thing we could do was to follow the current. It was such a terrifying experience for Luping, being squeezed mercilessly by the surge of people. When we finally got to the entrance, the attendant punched a small hole in our tickets.

The train slid in with a gust of wind. Through the train windows, I noticed there were many people aboard. Under the fluorescent light in the train, they looked like dead bodies preserved in formaldehyde. Passengers were not sure where the doors would be when the train stopped, so they started running alongside the train. Some were running toward the front of the train as if it were wartime and they were trying to take over the engine room. As the train finally came to a screeching halt, all the passengers pushed their way to the doors before they opened.

"Let the passengers get off first before boarding!" the attendant cried after she threw open the door nearest us.

We couldn't find any seats when we got onto the train. It was already full before it had arrived. Some passengers were standing in the corridors while others slept under the seats. Those of us who had just boarded rushed from cabin to cabin trying to find seats. It was a scene in which everyone seemed to be playing a joke on the newcomers, knowing that all the seats were taken but not bothering to tell us the truth, letting us find out on our own. They got satisfaction from watching us make fools of ourselves.

Finally, the train started moving, alleviating my anxiety. At first it moved very slowly then picked up speed. When it reached a certain speed, it maintained its rhythm. Wende rubbed his hand up and down his face several times as if he were washing his face without water. He had this habit of dry-washing his face, which I considered ominous. After what he had been through all night, he seemed a little relieved at that moment. There was a slight hint of that familiar contented look on his face that only I could recognize. He finally had a sense of closure. A bad result seemed better than no result at all.

In the early afternoon, next day, the train arrived in Tianjin. Passengers had started taking down their luggage from the overhead racks long before the train came to a standstill. Our family had to get off and change trains. Hearing the local accent gave me a strange feeling. We stayed in Tianjin for the night, and the next day boarded a train to Baodi County. By the time the train finally pulled into the Tianjin station, we were all extremely exhausted. It was quite some time after getting off that it occurred to me that I had left the thermos bottle behind — the very possession I had protected with my life the previous night. I talked about this incident with the family for many years. In fact, I just stopped talking about it in recent years because everyone was tired of hearing the story again and again! I guess it wasn't the story itself that had left such a deep impact on me, but the extreme circumstances in which it had happened.

PART III

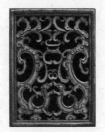

17

The Barefoot Doctor

"COME OVER HERE. Let me take a good look at you kids," Wende's blind sister yelled with a very high-pitched voice, using her plump hands to touch everyone from head to toe. She had come all the way from another village to greet us. When we arrived in the isolated village, everyone both young and old, came out to watch with great curiosity. The village head chased all the onlookers away.

"Fine-looking kids," Wende's sister said. "Luping's earlobes are quite thick — he will have good fortune when he grows up."

She was Wende's oldest sister. She had married at the tender age of seventeen. When she gave birth to her first baby, her husband asked for a divorce. During the first month after the childbirth, she cried constantly, and a month later she became blind. Wende was in the army at the time. When he heard the distressful news, he wrote several letters warning his sister's husband that he would hold him responsible if anything happened to his sister. That stopped the husband's talk of divorce.

When I finally met her, I was surprised at how white and fat the blind woman was. She ate and slept much of the time with never a worry on her mind. She often said: "If you don't see it, you don't worry about it."

Wende's second sister was married to a man in another village who later became a gang member. He was very abusive toward her. Her mother-in-law was a vicious old woman with only one eye, who constantly beat her up. When the mother-in-law smoked opium in bed, Wende's sister was force to kneel down and serve her.

In 1955, Wende's second sister was diagnosed with tuberculosis. Wende had wanted her to come to Shandong Province for treatment, so I had arranged a bed for her in the hospital. Unfortunately, her one-eyed mother-in-law and despicable husband hadn't allowed her to leave, and didn't seek treatment for her there either. For many years, half of Wende's wage had gone to his sister every month, and no one knew what they had done with it. In the meantime, I had mailed her a lot of antibiotic drugs. For a period of time, she had seemed better. But several years later, in 1962, we had received a letter informing us that she had passed away. She was only forty years old. I suspected that the malnutrition in the early sixties had also been part of the reason for her death.

Wende was actually from a fairly wealthy family before liberation. His father, Han Zhe, was a landlord. When he got married to Wende's mother, a landlord's daughter in a nearby village, their parents had an agreement that she would never go near three things: kitchen, well, and millstone. This meant she was the lady of the house, never having to lift a finger to do housework.

Later on, Wende's father plunged heavily into gambling, losing a great deal of money. To make things worse, he became ill. Doctors were constantly coming in and out, so often that the family would see one doctor heading out through the back door while one came in through the front. The family became more and more destitute, often going hungry. However, when Wende's mother stepped out, she remained well groomed. Every time people exchanged the conventional greeting, "Have you eaten?" with her, she immediately responded, "Yes." She liked to keep face.

It became necessary for her to handle all the household chores, from cooking in the kitchen and fetching water from the well, to grinding grain on the millstone. The agreement reached between their parents, which stated that she would not go near the "three things," was invalid. She was not only doing the "three things" but everything else as well. Shortly, the lady of the house developed a dark complexion from endless hours of labor under the intense sun, and a set of rough aching hands that were soaked in harsh lye soap on a regular basis. Wende's father died in 1936 when he was just forty years old.

Wende often mentioned how lucky his family was that his father had gambled their fortune away, otherwise they would have been labeled as landlords after liberation and become immediate targets of the revolution. During the land reform in the early fifties, the villagers held a mass rally in the old temple and beat the landlord from Shi clan to death. The landlord's belongings — land, houses, and furniture — were all distributed among the villagers. Wende's mother was allocated a house, but she was afraid to accept. She was such a timid person.

Initially, our family had to stay with Wende's brother, Han Guangde, until we found a place of our own. The interior settings of each house were the same throughout the village. When you walked in the front door, there were stoves on both sides that connected to the *kong* beds made of mud tiles. When meals were cooked in the stove, the *kong* beds would become toasty and comfortable on a cold night, but almost unbearable in summertime. We found that out for ourselves very soon.

Guangde's wife appeared polite toward me, but still held a grudge against me for the argument we'd had many years ago. In 1955, I had found a job for Guangde in Jiaonan County and his family lived with us for about six months. Occasionally I'd had some brushes with his wife. Now the tables had turned. To cook supper, she would use the stove connected to the *kong* bed that our whole family would sleep on that night. It was so unbearably hot that no one slept a wink all night.

The temperature soared to a scorching forty degrees outside, and, combined with the ovenlike bed, it was torture. The bed was so heated up that you could hatch eggs. For a moment I was sure that I heard the heat sizzling in the air. The window was completely sealed by white paper, and the door was blocked by a thick cotton curtain that wouldn't let in even the slightest breeze. I spent the entire night fanning the kids to cool them off.

Guangde's family slept in the cool *kong* bed on the opposite side of the hallway, with a bamboo screen hung comfortably over their doorway. Guangde's wife was probably having a good laugh.

"I can't take this anymore," I said. "I'll sleep in the yard."

"Just for my sake, please don't make a big deal out of this. It's a small village. Everyone will know in the morning and will laugh at us. Let's make do with it for the night and we'll think of something tomorrow, all right?" Wende said.

"Why do we care what they think? I can't sleep and the children can't sleep," I said.

"Lower your voice, we don't want them to hear."

The next morning, Wende invited the village head and some other important people for dinner, asking them to find us a place to live while we built our own house. Despite Wende's political problem, the villagers respected him and considered him to be a good and honest man. Old villagers all remembered what a good boy he had been before he left the village many years ago. Since they were relatives, the village chief called Wende "Uncle Five."

"Uncle Five, don't worry about it, I'll find a place for you," the village chief said.

At the time, Wende's elementary schoolteacher, who had introduced him to the Communist army, was also back in the village. "He is working under supervision in the village. There are two militiamen keeping an eye on him. Don't talk to him, Uncle Five, in case people gossip," the village chief said. He took a sip of liquor from the small cup and then put it down. "The policies of the Communist Party can change at any time," he added.

Wende and I were shocked at the way he talked so bluntly about the Communist Party. But I couldn't help thinking that there was some truth behind his ignorant comments. Many years later, I still pondered those words.

During the dinner, I also learned a great deal about the village from the chief. The village was called Xinwutun. Village names that included "tun" usually indicated that there had been troops stationed there in ancient times. The locals called the place in the west side of the village Qin City, even though it was just a hill in the middle of the sorghum field. The villagers believed that it was once a prosperous ancient town built by the first emperor Qin Shihuang's warriors, who had each brought a pocketful of soil from a faraway land to deposit there and make a grand palace. The soil in that area was black, while the rest remained yellow. From the front, it looked like a palace, and was believed to be where the emperor had temporarily stayed.

There was a strong belief among the villagers that treasure was buried underneath the ancient site. Adorned with grass and lots of thorny wild jujube trees, it was a home to an incredible number of different snakes — evidence of buried treasure that the snakes were safeguarding.

Legend had it that, a long time ago, a Taoist priest wearing a long gray robe had passed through the village. Supposedly, he had secretly told Wende's ancestor that there was a key in a gourd, and, if he cut it open when the fruit was ripe, the key inside could open Qin City, which contained enough treasure inside to last an eternity. The ancestor was ecstatic and took excellent care of the gourd, but as it grew larger and larger each day, he became increasingly impatient. Finally, unable to wait any longer, he chopped open the melon — only to find a key that had not yet matured. Filled with regret, he died shortly after.

There was another legend about Qin City: there was a street in the village called "Horse Escape." It was the only street that had a name, and there was a great tale behind it. For many days, Wende's ancestor noticed the water vat was emptying much quicker than usual. He suspected something was wrong and waited for a long time behind the door, until finally a beautiful horse appeared in the yard and headed straight for the water vat. The horse put its whole head down into the vat and started drinking thirstily. It only took a second for the creature to drain the vat. "That explains it!" the ancestor cried. He picked up a shovel and struck the horse. The horse shrieked and galloped away in the direction of Qin City. As it ran, a small piece of flesh fell from its thigh and turned into a chunk of pure gold. He never caught a glimpse of the mysterious horse ever again. Filled with regret, he died shortly after.

The villagers were convinced that things such as the horse were in fact treasure in disguise and that it came from Qin City. They also believed that when things became too old, they would magically come to life. Even a broom or a chair might have life of its own.

During the Great Leap Forward, villagers dug more than ten meters down into the hill of Qin City, discovering horse manure that was believed to date back a couple of thousand years to the period when the first emperor's warriors were stationed there. They also dug out a well-preserved mummy that took a long time to decompose.

For some reason, all the stories told by the villager chief ended with regrets. "If you don't have good fortune even when the fortune is right under your very eyes, you won't ever have it," he concluded and sipped his liquor thoughtfully.

The place the village chief found for us belonged to a family who had an extra room beside their home. Our whole family had to share the tiny room. Since the house faced west, in the hot summer afternoon, the sun would heat up the crowded space like an oven.

Xianping, at the age of fifteen, was denied admission to high school by the education bureau of Baodi County because of Wende's political problem. Xianping was not allowed to join the army either. Being a soldier was a very prestigious career at the time. It was probably the only way for the young people to ever get out of the countryside. Otherwise, there was no future. First, potential recruits were subjected to a very strict physical examination. Many young people had high blood pressure just because they were so nervous. It was said that drinking vinegar would help, so many desperate young people drank a whole bottle of it before the exam. Then there was a very thorough political background investigation. A recruiting officer really liked Xianping because he was strong and healthy. Of course, he failed to pass the high-standard political examination because of Wende's problem. "What a pity!" the officer said. I went to the commune to talk to a commissar in the armed forces department — a civilian organization that handled new army recruits — but it didn't work.

Wende went to the commune to plead for Xianping three times: once for him to be able to join the army, and twice concerning his education. All Wende's efforts failed. But since Xianping had graduated from junior high school, which was the highest academic attainment in the village, the village chief made him a teacher in the village elementary school. Since the motto may as well have been "the sky is high and the emperor is far away" in the isolated village, the chief didn't have to do everything according to the party's policy.

My daughter Yanping entered grade four in the village school. After school, she and Luping would go to the field to pick wild vegetables to feed the pig and rabbits.

It didn't take long for us to see that life in the countryside was really tough. We had to eat corn every day — cornbread, corn cereal, corn this, corn that. That's all we had. I even had to cook with corn stalks, which produced lots of smoke, making me cough and my eyes water. For cornbread, I first made the corn flour into dough, shaping it into foot-long loaves with my hands, and sticking them around the big pot one by one. When they were done, about one hour later, you could still clearly see the hand marks on the bread. The bottom side would be quite crispy.

The villagers all lived in adobe houses fenced with corn stalks. On the west side of the village, there was a pond where children swam and hunted for frogs while the women washed clothes and diapers on the shore. Guangde's second son was skilled in catching frogs with a long spear. The villagers had a habit of eating these slimy creatures. They were plentiful during the summer and often poked their heads out of the water to make "ribbit" sounds. The boy's spear was constructed out of a sorghum stalk and had a sharp metal point on one end. He would float the spear in front of him through the water as he approached the unsuspecting frogs. When he got close enough, he would strike and stab right through his prey.

On hot days, the middle-aged and old women would go topless in public or while working in the field. Even though it looked very strange to us, the conservative villagers never raised questions about the practice.

Villagers often dropped by to borrow things, much of which we never saw again. The most frequently borrowed item was the bike, since we were the only ones in the village to own one. Another item they liked to borrow was the radio. Some old people had never seen a radio before in their lives. They were all amazed by how the words and music flowed from the small box. Even the village chief admired it with awe.

Shortly after our arrival in the village, Wende had gathered some villagers to help him construct a house. After a few drinks at dinner, the workers promised that we would "see smoke coming out of the chimney after three days." In reality, it took several months to build the house, from preparing the necessary materials to the finish. But the time actually spent constructing the house was only twenty days.

When the time came to set the roof beam in place, all the relatives showed up. Wende had many relatives. There were only three main clans in the village. Han was the largest, and was divided into north Han and south Han. North Han was already out of *wufu* — five generations with the same blood relationship. Wende belonged to south Han. Those relationships were very confusing to me. I didn't know how to address them. Neither did my kids. Luping was only five years old and yet some of the relatives who were ten years older than him were calling him "grandfather."

"Why did that girl call me Little Grandpa?" Luping asked me.

"Go ask your father," I said.

"It's called *beifen*, seniority in a clan. It has nothing to do with your age," Wende said. "When in the village, do as the villagers do."

Putting on the roof beam was considered a very important event. It was a very thick, heavy beam placed in the middle of the bedroom ceiling. I didn't understand why it was necessary to use such a big beam, but the villagers were quite serious about it. By taking one look at the beam in your house, people could determine if you were rich or poor.

An old relative advised Wende that he should hire a good cook because it was an important event and there were so many guests, but I said I could do the cooking myself. "Do you know how to cook?" He laughed.

"Make sure you treat the carpenters and workers well, and don't offend anyone. Otherwise there will be a problem," the old relative said to us. He went on to tell a story about a family in the nearby village who offended the laborers when they built their house, the laborers made a little mud figure and hid it in the house to curse the family. The family ended up having one disaster after another. In the army Wende had been educated as an atheist and of course didn't believe in curses, but he really put a lot of effort into the event. He headed to town and bought fifty pounds of pork and several big fish.

As Wende took charge of the fire, I prepared several tasty dishes as well as eight pots of steamed buns, with more than ten big buns in each pot. The villagers were all amazed by it and never thought I could be such a good cook. During the banquet, Wende ran up and down to make sure that every worker was properly served, not daring to ignore anyone.

"Hey, how come they eat all the big fish?" Luping yelled.

"Don't talk so loud," I said, afraid the workers would hear him, causing bad luck.

Wende's brother Guangde never came to help with building the house. He said he was too busy, but I knew the real reason was that his wife didn't want him to come. Nevertheless, I saved some food for him. The next day, he showed up to check on the progress of the new house. I brought out the food I had saved for him to eat, but he refused it because he was afraid that his wife would find out and cause trouble.

The house was built in the same style as the rest of the houses in the village. We moved into our new home in early winter of 1970. It wasn't perfect but it was a place to call our own. The house, situated right on the edge of the village, allowed us an open view of the field. A little river flowed just beside the house. The next-door neighbor was very upset because the roof of our house was a little higher than theirs. The neighbor said that was bad feng shui for them.

As soon as we moved into the new house, we had a rat problem. The countryside was overrun by rats that were constantly stealing our food. I tried my best to hide food in the cupboard or in huge jars but they still managed to get into it. As a last resort, I placed the food into a basket, hanging it on the roof beam. This tactic also failed because the rats were somehow able to climb the rope. I started thinking that the pesky rodents were smarter than people. No sooner had I plugged one hole with mud when another would turn up somewhere else. The cat we raised had never caught a rat, even when it was hungry.

Even though the villagers had heard that I was a doctor, at first they had reservations about me. After we first got to the village, I had poured some water purifier into a nearby well — a water source for the whole village. The villagers all got scared silly and didn't go near the well for a long time because rumors had circulated that I had poisoned the water. They would rather walk a long distance to another village to get water. I had to explain to them that it was for their benefit. Slowly the villagers returned to the well.

Then they heard that I had cured the hookworm disease for one of Wende's relatives. The woman had already had the disease for over a year. She was very weak. Her face was pale and she lacked an appetite. The hookworm disease was quite common in the countryside, because peasants often went barefoot, or worked with mud barehanded. The worm would enter the body through the feet or hands, causing abdominal pain, loss of appetite, and anemia in cases of heavy infection. I suggested that the woman go to the county hospital to have some tests done. The test result confirmed my diagnosis. She took medication to get rid of the worms, and then slowly recovered with proper nutrition. After three months of treatment, the patient felt much better, her face gaining color and her appetite returning. She was very grateful to me. In the village, I had found four cases of hookworm disease.

The news spread fast, and after that the villagers flocked to me day and night. I treated them with the limited medicines I had brought with me to the countryside. Soon I received respect from the villagers. The village chief came to me and said: "Aunt, no matter what, you have great skill. They come to see you anyway. Why not open up a clinic, and you can earn some work points for grain?"

So I agreed and became a "barefoot doctor." That was what they called the country doctors who possessed minimal formal training, and limited equipment and supplies. Such doctors provided basic medical services, such as promoting hygiene and treating minor illness at the grassroots level. The barefoot doctor program was Mao's panacea for the peasants. The goal was to choose one peasant in each village with only junior high-school or high-school education, and train the person for a few months before he or she became a doctor. Mao believed practice made perfect. "There's no need to read so many books," Mao said. "The more you read, the more stupid you become." That was why universities across the country were shut down. The less the people knew the better. "Better red than an expert."

Traditional Chinese Medicine, including herbs and acupuncture, became a symbolic part of the barefoot doctor program. Mao believed it was safe, cheap, and "spiritually comforting." In other words, he provided peasants with a placebo. He knew that peasants had blind faith in mystical Chinese herbs, so he gave them what they wanted. It was a cheap solution since the barefoot doctors were not full-time. Barefoot doctors were still involved in farm work when not treating patients. Herbs were much cheaper than Western medicine, and were quite often grown by the barefoot doctors themselves in their own backyards. Diagnosing patients by feeling their pulses was obviously cheaper than laboratory tests, which required complicated equipment. Peasants were Mao's foundation, so he couldn't abandon them. Instead of establishing a real medical system and training more doctors, he chose the barefoot doctor program — another mass mobilization of peasants similar to the Great Leap Forward movement. This also showed Mao had no respect for science.

Before I came, there was already a barefoot doctor in the village. Villagers didn't seem to trust him. He could only treat the most common illnesses — colds, coughs, and diarrhea. During his three months of training, he had learned to use three prescriptions to treat the patients. When he used up his three formulas without seeing any effects, he would run out of ideas. He usually treated villagers who had tooth and stomach aches using acupuncture; it was much cheaper than any medicine. Villagers were afraid to see him because his acupuncture caused more pain than the illnesses themselves. On the surface, it seemed that the barefoot doctors had contributed a great deal to alleviate the peasants' suffering and to provide basic health care, but in my opinion, the program only masked the serious problems. It was just like the mobile medical team program — a mere political formality. I earned six work points a day, which provided our family with enough grain to eat. All the equipment I had could be put into a small case bearing a red cross. I was often disturbed at all hours of the night to see patients.

After we got a dog named Hali, the villagers coming to call on me at night would cautiously tiptoe around to the back of the house to avoid the animal. We got Hali when he was a pup. The first night, we left him in the yard. He was whining so loudly that we had to bring him inside, but he still didn't stop. Hali grew very quickly into a good guard dog. Every morning, he would follow Xianping and Yanping halfway to school and then run quickly home. When I set out at night to call on the sick, Hali would accompany me there and back, which made me feel very safe.

At seven o'clock one evening in early winter, shortly after we moved into our new house, a woman in the neighborhood knocked desperately on our door. Her seven-year-old son had suddenly become sick. When I arrived there, I found that the boy's lips and fingernails were darkened and he was struggling for breath. These were unmistakable symptoms of poisoning.

"What did the child eat?" I asked the mother.

"My neighbor gave me a bottle of medicine to treat my son's roundworms. He drank two spoons of the syrup around supper-time. He liked the taste of the sweet syrup and drank more later," the mother said. Roundworm disease was very common, especially among children in the countryside, where sanitation was poor.

"He's poisoned," I said. "Hurry, go to the commune hospital immediately." I was not equipped to handle it.

After the boy's father got a donkey cart ready, they headed to the commune hospital, which was ten miles away. The boy was already unconscious, his arms and legs flopping down limply in his mother's arms, just like a doll made of cloth.

At two o'clock in the early morning, I heard a cry of agony, faint at first, then becoming louder and louder as if someone was turning the volume up. I knew the child hadn't made it. I went over to see them.

"When we turned the corner near the hospital, my boy called, 'Mother.' That was his last word. He died before entering the emergency room," the mother told me. "Don't feel bad. The boy was probably from a noble family in a past life and we are not worthy of him, so he left." The sad woman was trying to comfort me.

They buried the boy in their backyard. He was their only son. The reason they hadn't come to me for help when the boy first had stomach pain from roundworms was because the boy's father had taken part in the construction of our new house, and, for some unknown reason, was offended. After the boy's death, they regretted not having sought me out for help.

They also had a fourteen-year-old daughter who had had infantile paralysis, leaving her with a limp. Infantile paralysis, also called polio, is a communicable disease caused by a viral infection, affecting the whole body including the muscles and nerves. Severe cases may cause permanent paralysis, even death. It was once a worldwide epidemic affecting mostly infants and children. There was no vaccine for the disease available when the girl was young.

Two days after the boy's death, the neighbor who gave the family the medicine was outraged with me because even though I didn't blame him for the boy's death I was the one who had said the boy was poisoned. He came over to our place to pick a fight and created a big stir. All the villagers came to gawk.

"I didn't make it up," I said. "There is a hospital record."

"I know your political background. Are you staging a comeback? You should be careful!" he threatened me and Wende. I realized that even in a small village there was political struggle.

The Chinese New Year was approaching and I was busier than ever. Around nine o'clock on a cold evening, I heard Hali bark. An old man showed up with his nineteen-year-old son who was suffering from severe stomach pain. I suspected that he had intussusception, a condition that occurs when a portion of the bowel folds in on itself, resulting in decreased blood supply of the involved segment. Early diagnosis and treatment could salvage the boy's bowel.

"Go to the commune hospital immediately," I said. "He needs surgery."

They hurried off to the commune hospital. At midnight, I heard Hali bark. The father and son came calling on me again. This time the son had a very high fever and unbearable pain in the stomach. Apparently the hospital hadn't performed an operation on him but instead had just sent him home with some painkillers. The patient's father went down on his knees and pleaded to me. "I beg you to save my son, grandmother!" According to seniority in the Han clan, I was the old man's grandmother. I accompanied the patient to the commune hospital.

"Why didn't you come earlier?" the doctor said. Instead of

admitting his mistake, he accused the patient.

They finally operated on the young man, cutting off about fourteen inches of intestine, which could have been avoided if they had operated on the young man sooner. That was the way they treated the peasants. The father and son didn't dare to talk back. They looked as if they had committed a crime. I had seen doctors treat patients like this when I worked in the hospital and always felt sympathetic toward the poor peasants. Now I was one of them, so I knew exactly how they felt.

18

Going to Beijing

On New Year's Eve, I was preparing food for the next few days. I was raised to believe that people were not supposed to cook at the beginning of the New Year. That would bring bad luck and things could go wrong for the whole year. Like my mother, I also watched the kids carefully to make sure that they wouldn't say anything stupid.

At suppertime, Wende brought some chopsticks to the table. I counted them and became upset. "I told you so many times, don't bring out the chopsticks in odd numbers — it's very ominous. They should always be in even numbers," I scolded. As usual, I was met with his silence, which was worse than an argument.

For some reason, the holiday put Wende into a bad mood. He became anxious and irritated very easily. Those last few years, he was never happy during the holidays. On the surface he appeared calm and even-tempered. However, he became a completely different person when the New Year came. He was dissatisfied with everything: the furniture was in the wrong place, the children were talking too loudly, or dinner was twenty minutes late, even though he was not hungry and had nothing urgent to do afterward. Right after the holiday, he would return to normal again. It was as if he was glad that the holiday was over so he could get on with his life.

During the New Year, Wende invited over his old fellow-villager who had come back from Beijing. He brought back many pieces of "grapevine news," which isolated villagers could never otherwise have access to. He was surprised by the way Wende had been treated by the army and didn't think it was justified. That was when I conceived the idea of going to Beijing to appeal the army's verdict on Wende's case. The old fellow-villager invited me to stay at his place if I decided to go to Beijing, but he cautioned me that it was not easy to get there, because a person had to have a permit from the authorities to enter Beijing.

"No, it's out of the question," Wende said firmly when I talked to him about my intention.

"Why not?" I said. "What do we have to lose?"

"Things could get worse. Let sleeping dogs lie. We have everything we need here; what more could we ask for? We should consider ourselves lucky to still be alive. Besides, what result can you hope to achieve? There's already a conclusion," he said.

"Our children can't stay in the countryside their entire lives. There's no future for them here. Look, Xianping couldn't go to high school or join the army because of your political problem. I looked at his diary the other day. It made me so sad. He's so young but has had so many setbacks. He's really frustrated. As a parent I feel guilty. Even if there is a very small chance, I think we should try our best," I said.

"How could the Communist Party make a mistake? If there was a mistake made, they will correct it. We don't need to appeal, we can just wait," Wende said.

"How long are we going to wait? Our children are growing up. We have to think of them."

When the spring came, Wende planted numerous fruit trees, such as apple, peach and pear, in our front yard and backyard. Very serious about his new venture, he went to the town and bought some garden tools. He became a farmer, heading out every morning with a hoe on his shoulder and returning in the evening. He always brought back some grasshoppers to feed the chicken. He seemed content with the situation. He always said: "Contentment brings happiness." Well, judging by the thick and strong roof beam in the house that he built, I realized that he was determined to stay in the countryside for the rest of his life. I couldn't really blame him for that because I knew he had suffered a lot, but I had to consider our children's future.

In April of 1971, I decide to make the trip to Beijing. It was hard to obtain a leave from the village chief, so I pretended to have a health problem that would require me to go to Beijing for a checkup.

"You look healthy to me, Aunt," he said. "You're a doctor yourself, why do you have to go to see a doctor?"

"I can't treat myself," I said to him.

"I don't mind giving you a leave. It's just that people will gossip."

The village chief finally agreed. Coincidentally, the person in charge of purchasing goods for the village was also going to Beijing. I convinced him to take me with him, since he had a permit to enter Beijing. When I got to Beijing, Wende's fellow-villager arranged a one-month temporary *hukou* — residence registration — for me at the local police station. As an added benefit, I was allotted one pound of canola oil for cooking, and a coupon good for a five-foot piece of cloth for making clothes. These everyday items were all strictly rationed.

The next morning, I walked to the reception office of the State Council on Taiping Street. The entrance was extremely small in comparison to the towering red walls surrounding the office. On the first day, I wasn't even able to get past the entrance. It was swarming with visitors. There was a long lineup outside the office. Some visitors were sleeping at the foot of the high wall. Since there were five or six hundred people visiting the government office each day, I had to write an application first, and wait for a week before I could see anyone.

A week later, I finally had a chance to talk to a naval officer whose rank was impossible to tell because of the simplified army uniform. I told him the whole story.

"My husband was treated unjustly," I explained to the officer.

"If everything you've told me is true, then maybe your husband's case was handled incorrectly," the officer said. "But there's nothing we can do about it. You have to go to the people who directly handled the case. Your husband should write a detailed report and take it to the Jinan Military District. Ask for Commander Yang. Don't come here anymore. There's nothing we can do about it."

That was the end of the conversation. However, I felt I hadn't made the trip for nothing because I had received advice from the central government. I felt as if I were bearing the "emperor's sword," a symbol of discretionary power.

Twenty days later, I returned home to find Wende still with blisters on his lips that had been caused by anxiety. As if waiting for something to go wrong, he asked me about everything except the result of the trip.

"There's hope," I said. "There's nothing they can do, but they told me that you should write a report and take it to Commander Yang of the Jinan Military Region. You don't need to do anything around the house. Just concentrate on writing the report. I will take care of everything."

Wende refused to write the report.

"Don't you feel they treated you unjustly?" I asked him.

"Yes, I do, but if the party made a mistake, they will correct it," he said.

Next day, Yanping and Luping played with the checkers I had brought back from Beijing and got into a fight. Luping lost the game and went into the yard to destroy the flowers his sister had planted. Her hobby was to plant flowers and she was very dedicated to it. "Damn kids! Don't play anymore," Wende said. He got angry and threw the checkerboard across the room. Yanping and Luping spent the rest of the day hunting in every corner for the missing pieces.

"We've just gotten used to the daily life here. I know it's not perfect, but at least it's calm. Why can't you leave well enough alone?" Wende said to me.

"Now it's all my fault. You got us into this mess. I should've never come to this place with you. What was I thinking?" I said angrily. Later, of course, I regretted what I had said.

I also brought back a box of pastries that were famous in Beijing. Even before I opened the box, the children were tempted by the sight of the oil showing through from the delicious sweets inside. That was a real treat for kids who had only been chewing on cornbread for a couple of years. I told them that they could have just a little each time and carefully hid the box where they couldn't find it. The children pestered me about it all the time. Days later, when I finally agreed to let them have some, I found to my surprise that the desserts were all gone. The hole in the box indicted that rats had gotten into it. "Those damn rats, you just can't hide anything from them," I said. I felt very bad about it because I had denied the children the chance to enjoy them. We then started another futile campaign to get rid of those pests.

I couldn't convince Wende to write the report no matter how hard I tried. By fall, he was too busy with the harvest to write anything. As I've probably made clear, corn was the main staple in the villagers' diet. First, the corn was picked, then the stalks were cut with sickles. After the corn dried, our whole family went to earn some extra work points by removing every kernel of corn manually; the work made our hands blistered and sore.

By the end of the year, Wende finally yielded to my protests and started writing. He always saved his documents and letters. Therefore, all he needed to do was put his material together, make a few changes, and add some information. Wende didn't say much; he was able to express himself better through writing. He first wrote a draft, then made a clean copy without a single error. When he finished his writing, it was already approaching the New Year. It was a long letter.

> *Dear leaders of the Party Committee of the Military Region,*
>
> *I was the former head of the supply department of the 601 Regiment, 201 Division of 67 Army. In July of 1970, during the Cleanse the Class Ranks, I was purged from the army and party and sent to my hometown due to questions about my personal history. I was in shock about the outcome and I have been very frustrated ever since. However, I have no other choice but to obey. I have the following opinions which I would like to present to the Party Committee. Needless to say, these are all from my own personal point of view. I sincerely hope that the Party Committee will deal with the matter according to our party's policy.*
>
> *I had risked my life working underground for the Communists before liberation. If I was caught by the enemy, there was no doubt that I would have been tortured and killed. During the Cleanse the Class Ranks, the 67 Army Party Committee concluded I was a historical counter-revolutionary. I couldn't comprehend this. I was always very strict with myself. During the Civil War, some comrades in my squad deserted the army, but I followed Chairman Mao's instruction and "carried the revolution to the end." During the War to Resist America and Aid Korea, I sacrificed my own interest by postponing my marriage and giving up the*

*thought of going home to attend my mother's funeral. I have
stood up to a severe test and worked even harder, so my work
was not affected in any way. Because of that, I was praised by
the party and won a third-class merit citation. Talking about
standing the test, I have withstood for twenty-five years. I am
faithful to the revolution, not half-heartedly, and don't have
any "ulterior motives." It is very difficult for me to accept the
verdict that I "infiltrated" the army and party. I don't know if
this is the central government's policy. Chairman Mao had
pointed out that the party should "narrow the scope of
purging and expand the scope of education."*

*My problem has directly affected my wife and children.
My wife Li Qunying joined the army in 1945 and was transferred to the local hospital in 1955. She often gave up the
weekends and holidays to participate in the socialist con-
structions. Isn't all this genuinely for the revolution, or what?
Jiaonan County forced her to resign from her job and the
party simply because she refused to divorce me. Before
coming to the countryside, I pleaded to the army to let her
continue her work in the hospital, but even this reasonable
request was denied. My son Xianping wanted to go to school,
but was denied. I have contacted the county and commune
many times concerning this matter, but was disappointed.
My son cried for several nights. Being parents, we felt heartbroken. . . .*

Revolutionary Salutations!
Han Wende
April 10, 1972

In April of 1972, I took the report and went to Jinan, the capital city of Shandong Province, where the Jinan Military Region
headquarters was located. I changed trains in Tianjin, and
arrived in Jinan in the afternoon of the next day. It was still
quite cold and I was wearing a heavy sweater.

After arriving at the office of the Jinan Military Region, I asked for Commander Yang. The receptionist looked at me from the corner of his eyes. "Who do you think you are? Do you have any idea who Commander Yang is? You think you can just see him anytime you want?" he said sarcastically.

"The officer from the State Council in Beijing told me to see him," I said, taking out the "emperor's sword."

It seemed to work. The receptionist made a phone call, and, a short while later, an official came out from the inner room and introduced himself as the chief of staff.

"Commander Yang is not in. You can talk to me about it," he said to me.

After I told him the whole story, the officer said: "Leave the document with me and go home to wait. We'll let you know our decision."

When I came out of the office, it was already evening. I returned to the station in the hope of catching the train home but there were none at that hour. I had no money to stay in a hotel so I tried to sleep on the bench in the waiting hall. The police came by to check for valid tickets and showed the door to anyone who didn't have one. I wandered aimlessly for hours in the street until my knees started aching. I had gotten arthritis during the torturous army life in the Korean War. Finally, I noticed a lighted sign that said "Public Bathhouse."

The bathhouse bustled with customers during the day, but at night after nine o'clock it was closed to bathers and open to those who required a cheap bed for the night. Each bed was separated by a wooden partition. It was difficult to sleep deeply because of the fleas crawling all over me. At midnight, I woke up disoriented and couldn't figure out where I was.

"It's time to get up!" someone yelled and dazzling bright lights hurt my eyes.

I looked at my watch and realized it was only five in the morning. It was still dark outside. People's voices and the sound of coughing began to filter in from outside, along with the rustle of big bamboo brooms as people swept the yard. The guests were told to pack. Bathhouse workers were already getting the place cleaned up and prepared for that day's opening. All the guests had risen. The chaotic scene reminded me of an emergency assembly when I was in the army.

I came back home and waited and waited. But after several months I still hadn't heard anything from the Jinan Military District. I had been hopeful at first, but as time dragged on, my patience wore thin.

A few months later, we received a letter from Wende's old comrade Shouyi who was then living in the city of Tangshan, not far from Beijing. I thought we had been forgotten by the outside world up until then. During that time, we never received letters. Who would dare write to a counter-revolutionary family? Letters could be used as "black words on white paper" — evidence if something went wrong. No one wanted to risk getting into such serious trouble. Just like the old proverb warns: "The wise man protects himself." But Shouyi wasn't a wise man. He was born in Sanhe County, an area known for its fools. The letter was very short.

> According to landlord's information, there are some policy changes. There are new policies concerning Wende's problem. His case was handled incorrectly.

After reading the letter, we were all confused by the phrase "according to landlord's information." Landlords were the target of the revolution. Who would want to have anything to do with them? How could he get information from a landlord? Wende handed the letter to me, and I handed it back to him. We read it numerous times, but still couldn't make heads or tails of it. Finally, after contemplating it the whole night, we figured out that it was a misspelling. Shouyi meant to say "according to dependable information." Because he didn't know how to spell the words, he replaced them with some similar sounding and easily spelled words. It became a standing joke in my family. "He could have got into serious trouble," Wende said. He didn't think it was a funny matter at all. After reading it, he burned the letter in the stove.

In July, I decided to make another trip to Beijing. On my previous trip, I went to the State Council. This time I wanted to try my luck at the General Political Department. Wende wasn't strongly against the idea this time, even though he wasn't enthusiastic about it. "I have an old comrade who worked in the General Political Department. His name is Wu Zhijian. I knew him when we worked together at the bomb factory when I'd just joined the army. We were very good friends, and, after I left the factory, we wrote to each other quite often." He handed me a letter that was written by the old comrade bearing his address. "Go to find him and he may be able to help."

The trip was much more complex than the first. Since I didn't have a permit to enter Beijing, I had no choice but to buy a ticket to Tushan County. From there, I purchased a ticket to Tongxian County where there were regular buses to Beijing city center every half an hour. I stayed with Wende's fellow-villager and I was completely shocked and bewildered to learn of Lin Biao's downfall. Shouyi's dependable information was in fact based on the rumor of Lin Biao's downfall, an event that we were kept in the dark about for almost a year. In the previous September, Lin Biao, the vice chairman and "the dearest and closest comrade of Chairman Mao," along with his wife and son, had tried to flee to the Soviet Union after an unsuccessful coup attempt. They were all killed when their plane ran out of fuel, crashing in Mongolia. It was almost a year before the official news of his attempted coup and tragic demise began to be made public. After 1969, Chairman Mao finally became aware of the political ambition of Lin Biao. As a result, Lin was losing Mao's favor and his position began to deteriorate.

"Do you know how Lin Biao died?" the old fellow-villager said mysteriously. "His plane didn't run out of fuel — it was shot down by a missile. How could Chairman Mao let such an important official escape to the Soviet Union? Chairman Mao knew about Lin Biao's plot from the very beginning and he just wanted to see how far Lin Biao would go." That was the most popular "grapevine news" at the time. People were still hush-hush about the Lin Biao incident. His death was a mystery. The official story was that the plane ran out of fuel, but there were many other speculations surrounding it. Some said that a time bomb placed on-board brought down the plane while others claimed that it was shot down by the Soviet Union. The most conflicting theory came when the Soviet experts who inspected the crash scene concluded that the plane was in fact on its way back to China when it crashed.

According to the fellow-villager, even U.S. President Nixon, who visited China on his historical trip in February 1972, was kept in the dark. He couldn't find the second-in-charge Lin Biao, who always followed Mao loyally around, waving Mao's Little Red Book in his hand.

"Where is your vice-chairman?" he asked Mao, but never got a satisfactory answer.

In a way some of these rumors sounded comic but they showed that people lacked confidence in the official news. After Lin Biao's downfall, people began to have doubts about things they were told. They didn't know what to believe any-more. Since Lin Biao was single-handedly responsible for Mao's personal cult, in some ways his death marked the beginning of the end of Mao worship.

Whatever happened to Lin Biao, it represented a new hope for my family. I got up early the next morning and headed to the General Political Department. Walking down the busy streets in Beijing, I could feel the uncertain change in the air. The bells of the bicycles sounded extremely clear in the early morning. When the red light came on at the intersection, people on bicycles stopped, and gradually gathered into a dark mass. When the light turned green, the wave of bicycles rushed forward like a dam suddenly bursting.

The General Political Department, also surrounded by towering red walls, was not too far from the reception office of the State Council I had visited on my previous trip. The place was also swarming with people. Outside the office, at least thirty visitors were waiting. Inside, a fairly high brick wall separated the officers from the visitors. There were six officers sitting in a row, talking to the visitors. Ten armed soldiers were guarding the office, inside and outside. While I registered and waited for my name to be called, I heard a desperate person cursing the officers loudly, and he was soon hauled away by the guards.

When I finally heard my name called and approached the counter, I found that the wall was much higher than I had thought. It was almost to my neck. If I was just a little bit shorter, I wouldn't have been able to see the officer on the other side. The uniformed officer was a middle-aged woman with a Hebei accent. The whole interview lasted less than ten minutes.

"It was Liu Shaoqi's policy when your husband joined the army. Now with him brought down, there's no way we could reverse the verdict," the officer said, rudely interrupting me in the middle of my speech. She spoke in a firm, cold tone to indicate that she was not willing to listen or answer any questions.

"My husband has devoted twenty-five years to the country and this is the way you treat him? Where's the justice?" I said desperately. She and the other officers just laughed and mocked me.

I came out of the office and set out to find Wende's old comrade, the last gleam of hope. He lived not too far away from the General Political Department. It didn't take long for me to find him by following the residential address on the envelope. I introduced myself when he opened the door halfway.

"I don't know anyone named Han Wende," he said.

I took out the letter to show him. "Did you write this letter?" I asked him.

"No. I didn't write the letter."

"But it has your signature on it, and it is dated just two years ago when Wende was still in the army. How can you deny it?"

"No. I don't know him," he said, and shut the door in my face.

19

REHABILITATION

LUPING STARTED SCHOOL at the age of seven in the fall of 1972. The school was at the old temple in the village. After liberation, religion was forbidden and all idols of deities in the temple were replaced with Chairman Mao's pictures.

Classroom space was extremely limited and there were not enough teachers, so one teacher had to teach two grades in a single classroom. The room was divided down the middle with grade one on one side and grade two on the other. The teacher would tell the grade one students to study by themselves while he was teaching grade two and vice versa. In the first class, Luping learned how to write "Long live Chairman Mao," and he came home to show me.

Since there was only an elementary school in the village, Yanping had to walk several miles a day to reach the junior high school in the commune. She had to rise quite early and often got back home after dark. We worried every time she returned home late. Another girl from the village also attended the same school so they always walked together. One evening, Yanping failed to return after seven o'clock. We were worried sick. I went to the other girl's family and found that she hadn't come home either, but her parents didn't seem worried at all. Wende set out immediately to look for Yanping on the road leading from the village. I kept my ears fixed on that road. My eyesight was poor but my ears were sharp.

About an hour later, to my relief, I heard them talking in the distance.

The distance of the school and the anxiety that this caused were among the many difficulties that we faced every day of our lives in the village.

In late fall, they arranged a room for me in the temple to set up a clinic and also provided me with some money to buy medicine and equipment. Before I just had a box to store my medicine and equipment, but now I had a clinic with a desk, a bed, and a medicine shelf. I started work at eight every morning, and went home at five or six in the afternoon. The villagers usually didn't have to go to the commune hospital miles away.

Just a few days after the clinic was set up, Wende's elementary teacher, who had introduced him to the Communist army, came to see me. He had diarrhea. Usually there were two militiamen watching him, but that day he came alone. I didn't know the whole story of Wende's history so I asked him about it.

"Don't worry. I won't tell anyone," I said to him.

He looked around to make sure nobody was listening. "No one knows Wende better than I do," he whispered. "He's a good boy. I knew him from a very young age." He told me the whole story. Wende rarely spoke about his past. I received more information about him from his teacher and relatives than from himself.

On a warm day in June 1973, I was picking peaches in the yard. The second year after Wende had planted them, the fruit trees had yielded fruit. The big peaches looked delicious but tasted very sour. We also planted all kinds of vegetables, like potatoes, tomatoes, and cucumbers. We became self-sufficient.

On this particular day, two uniformed army officers came into the yard. They were from the 201 Division of the 67 Army. The officials admitted that they had mistreated Wende, but they blamed everything on Lin Biao. They restored Wende's reputation in the army, and his party membership. Wende was so excited and grateful that he shouted: "Long live Chairman Mao! Long live Chairman Mao!"

After the demise of Lin Biao in 1971, some officials who had been persecuted during the earlier stage of the Cultural Revolution were rehabilitated. Among them was Deng Xiaoping, who was reappointed as vice premier in April 1973.

The so-called rehabilitation turned out to be in name only. Wende was not allowed to go back to the army and wear the uniform. Instead, he was forced to retire at the age of forty-six. The army had no intention of using him again. He had pleaded with the army many times to let him resume his previous work, but each time he was denied. At that point, he didn't want to push his luck, and had no choice but to accept their decision. Later, Wende's schoolteacher was also rehabilitated. He resumed his job in Tianjin, and was doing quite well the last time I heard.

Even though Wende's verdict was reversed, I still experienced problems with my work. Jiaonan County Hospital, where I had worked before, refused to take me back. An officer from the 201 Division went to the local government but it didn't solve the problem. "It was the army's fault because you were the one who convinced us to expel Li Qunying from the hospital. You can't put someone back whenever you want. We have procedures," they told the army officer.

The second time, two officers from the army went. This time, the officials from the local government said they would have to discuss the matter. With that promise, the army informed me that I could go back to work. When I took a train ride to Jiaonan and reported to the local government office, they told me that the government hadn't reached an agreement with the army at all. After I got back home, Wende wrote a letter to the party committee of the 201 Division and the 67 Army:

> Because of my political problem, my son Xianping is not allowed to receive education and not allowed to join the army. Why isn't my wife Li Qunying allowed to work? At the beginning, the party spent so much time and effort to deal with my case in the study group. But when the time came to reverse the verdict, everything was done in an oversimplified way. There is no painstaking ideological work or compensation for our feelings. There are too many actual problems waiting to be solved.

I was like a beach ball being kicked back and forth between the army and the local government. The third time, the 201 Division and the 67 Army sent two officers to the local government with a letter from the party committee of the 67 Army to apologize to the local government. Only then did they agree to let me go back to work.

Our family left the village at the end of December 1973 and celebrated the New Year of 1974 in a guest house of 201 Division in Jiaoxian County. We went to a photo studio and had a rare family picture taken. Everyone was wearing heavy winter clothes, looking cold and disoriented.

We had no choice but to leave our dog Hali behind because pets were not allowed on the train, and forbidden in urban areas. All these years I've felt guilty about it. We betrayed Hali.

I have never returned to the village since. About twenty years after we'd gone, I heard a freak story about our old house. Out of the blue, the thick roof beam, which seemed strong enough to last for a hundred years, had one day suddenly broken without any warning. Villagers believed it was a very ominous sign. Only a few months later, one of Guangde's daughters-in-law, who lived in the old house, died of some sort of disease. The house was torn down shortly after.

We stayed in the guest house of 201 Division in Jiaoxian for four days until our belongings arrived at the train station. Then the army sent a truck to haul our family and possessions to my new workplace. I didn't go back to the hospital where I had worked before. Instead they sent me to a hospital in a small hilly town called Luwong Commune, in Shandong Province. When we arrived, we unwrapped the well-packed wooden boxes — our major assets. Even though they had undergone so many handlings, they still remained in fairly good condition. There were now only six of them left, down from the original eight.

Next, it was crucial to set up the cast-iron stove to keep warm in the cold winter and to cook meals. It didn't take long to assemble the parts of the stove and stovepipes. When the lumps of coal started to burn, the stove gave out a puff after puff of choking black smoke, soon followed by a roaring fire that immediately made the side of the stove, and the bottom part of the pipe, red. It heated up the entire apartment and gave us a nice homey feeling after our long journey. By placing or removing the three cast-iron rings on top of the stove, the appliance would fit different sizes of cooking pots and pans. Over time, ashes would build up in the stovepipes and Wende would take them apart, clean them by gently tapping, and then re-assemble. As a precaution, the fire had to be exterminated before bedtime because many people died each year from odorless carbon monoxide.

Right after we settled in, a new problem arose. My son Xianping's *hukou*, the residence registration, remained in the village. The reason given was that he was already eighteen and his residence registration couldn't be transferred. The residence registration was either urban or rural. With a rural *hukou* there was no chance of finding a job in the city. At once, Wende developed blisters on his lips. He couldn't eat or sleep.

In early 1974, I set out again to the 201 Division, which was stationed in Jiaoxian.

"No. It can't be done, because your son is already eighteen. If a child is under eighteen, he can be registered under the parents' name, but as soon as he turns eighteen, he has to have his own *hukou*. And that can't be transferred easily. That's the policy," a young officer said.

"I understand it is the policy, but my son Xianping went to the countryside because of his father's political problem. Now that his father's verdict has been reversed, my son's problem should also be solved," I said.

"No, we have to do everything according to our party's policy," the officer said.

"Because of the army's mistake, my son lost the opportunity to go to school and to join the army. Now he has to stay in the countryside for the rest of his life and won't be able to find a job. All these years I have appealed so many times to the central government in Beijing and to the army in Jinan. For what? For my children! And this is the result?" I said.

Finally, I lost my temper, jumped up, and flipped the desk over. The ink spilled onto the floor and paper scattered everywhere. At first they were astonished. Then the officer said: "Don't do anything, leave everything the way it is. This is a crime scene now."

"Let me tell you something," I said to the young officer. "When I joined the army, you were still wearing diapers. So don't talk to me that way."

A senior officer came out from the inner room. "This is not the way to solve a problem. Why not leave the matter with me, and I'll look into it. Go home and wait," he said in a sympathetic tone.

It took several months before Xianping's *hukou* was transferred. In December, he was allotted a job in Jiaonan Tractor Repair Station, which he didn't care for. But at that time he was already too old to resume school, and had never learned any usable skills. Even though he did try hard to educate himself, it could not make up for the education he had missed.

Yanping and Luping resumed school, where most students were country kids and hated children who "ate the government's grain." Even the teachers, who were mostly from the countryside, abused Luping physically and verbally. I went to the school to protest a couple of times but only made the matter worse.

Luwong was one of the poorest places in Shandong Peninsula, where peasants ate moldy sweet potato chips all year round and wore thin, patched clothes during the bitter winter. The students from the countryside often wiped their noses with their sleeves, and, over time, their sleeves got so shiny that a match could be lit on them. Many children never had enough to eat. Some kids made a habit of stealing the compressed pig feed that was made of bean by-products and brought it to school to chew on. Luping came home one day and asked me for some money. I asked him what it was for, and he told me that one of his classmates needed it to buy medicine for his sick mother. It was very generous of him to do that.

Each week there were "labor classes," in which all the students participated in manual labor. The school kids never really had much of a summer vacation because they had to labor in the fields with the villagers. When the villagers cut the wheat, the children's duty was to pick up loose ears. After the wheat was cut, the stalks left protruding from the ground were sharp, like knives. Yanping and Luping's feet were slashed numerous times even when they were wearing sandals. It didn't bother the country kids, who all ran around barefoot.

The villagers worked very hard, the sweat and dust soaking into their clothes, white alkaline visible on their backs. If there was a drought, students had to assist the peasants in watering crops. Kids had to carry water from far away, using buckets and wash basins. Near the end of the "summer holiday," the kids would collect the insects that were destroying the corn crops. The corn leaves often cut into their arms and the sweat would cause the cuts to sting painfully.

In the fall, the kids would be given a "fall holiday" to help the peasants harvest sweet potato and cut them into chips. In wintertime, students were sent by the school to search the mountains for pine cones in order to heat up the classroom. I wonder what else the kids learned in that school besides manual labor.

Our struggle was far from over. The political situation was almost identical to what it was before we went to the country-side. People went to meetings every evening, got up at five in the morning to sweep the yards, and were still on the lookout for adulterers. I resumed my work as a physician in the Internal Medicine Department. Even though Wende and I had decent wages and life had improved enough that we didn't have to eat corn every day, Wende was even more depressed. Because he was forced into retirement at the age of forty-six, he had nothing to do each day besides read the newspaper and pace around the small apartment. He was not a social person and rarely went out. Even though we were "liberated" politically, our overall life hadn't changed much. Five of us were cramped into the one-bedroom-and-living-room apartment while the children were all growing up. There was a rule at the time that officials with Wende's rank were allowed to live in mid-sized cities, which had better living conditions. He was also eligible for a bigger apartment. He went to ask the army about this matter many times but didn't achieve any results. He pursued it for many years — until the day he died.

"What's the big deal?" I said. "As long as we have a place to live." I tried to comfort him.

"Now I've become a housewife," he said. I understood how he felt. Despite the fact that he had dedicated his whole life to the army and was still in his best years, he was not allowed to work. He especially hated the cooking part, a duty he had to take on while I was working. It really hurt the man's self-esteem.

20

Seeing Chairman Mao Again

In the summer of 1975, I was transferred to another small hilly town called Dachang Commune, Shandong Province. There was only a wall that separated our residential compound and the hospital wards. When someone died in the wards, residents could clearly hear people crying. A few days after I started work at the new hospital, I saw a peasant who was dead on arrival in the emergency room. He was fatally injured in a blast while working in a quarry where explosives were often used. When he was hauled to the hospital on a small tractor, he was already dead, blood dripping down the trunk of the vehicle. Together with another doctor, I took the body to the morgue positioned at the gate of the hospital. The next day, the family of the deceased, relatives, and even neighbors came to say farewell. It was calm at first, but right after the group had gathered, the wailing suddenly broke out. It didn't happen spontaneously, but was more staged, so it sounded fake and stylized, like an act in a local opera. These sorts of wailing sessions were a very common custom in the countryside. Some people attended just to receive a free meal afterward.

In the fall of 1975, many cases of hemorrhagic fever were found in the area. During the Korean War, I had seen this rodent-transmitted disease that caused symptoms such as fever, bleeding from many sites on the body, and kidney failure

— but I didn't expect to find it there two decades later. The treatment included injections of hormone and glucose. In the two-month period, I had found about twenty patients with this disease. Unlike the cases I had encountered during the Korean War, the fatality rate at this time was low, due to the proper treatment in the hospital. This disease can still be found today in some areas of China.

On a hot night in July of 1976, a year after I was transferred to Dachang hospital, I was on my night shift in the emergency room. Since there were no patients at the time, I took a rest on a bed in which many patients had died. It didn't bother me so much because I had seen too many people die. Just a few days earlier, there was a peasant woman who had died on that very emergency bed. She had committed suicide by drinking pesticide after a domestic dispute. I couldn't save her even after taking all necessary measures. Cases like these were very common. Around midnight, I dosed off and had a terrifying dream. I was carrying a deceased patient to the morgue, when the corpse suddenly rose up and started chasing me. As hard as I tried, I couldn't get myself to run any faster. I woke up sweating heavily, my heart racing. Being chased was a re-occurring dream that I often had.

At midnight, I was woken by constant footsteps in the hallway. I thought it could be a patient coming in. I got up to check but there was no patient. It was the old and skinny pharmacist walking back and forth in the hallway, smoking a pipe. He was also on duty in the pharmacy, which was on the opposite side of the emergency room. The unique odor of the disinfectant permeated the long corridor. At intervals along the ceiling, lights glowed dimly, except for the one that had burnt out and left that area of the hallway in shadow.

"Why don't you sleep at this hour?" I asked the pharmacist curiously.

"I can't sleep. There seem to be rats in the pharmacy. The medicine bottles were rattling," he said. "Maybe because some traditional Chinese medicine uses grain as an ingredient. That may have attracted rats."

One hour later, for the second time, I was woken up. It was the old pharmacist again. Every time he finished one pipe, he would knock his pipe against the concrete floor to empty the ashes, then reload the tobacco.

"I can't sleep. There are noises," he said.

It was a very strange night. The next morning we heard the news that an earthquake had rocked Tangshan City where Wende's old comrade Shouyi lived, but details about the full extent of the disaster were never released. Many years passed before a government document estimated the death toll at 600,000 in a major quake, which measured 8.3 on the Richter scale. The quake also shook Tianjin and Beijing. It was unbelievable that the old pharmacist had felt something even though Tangshan was more than three hundred miles away.

It wasn't long before Wende received a letter from his friend and learned that his favorite daughter had been killed in the devastating quake. Wende decided to pay Shouyi a visit. I was against the idea because of the fact that it remained very dangerous there. Aftershocks were still occurring after the big quake. However, Wende was quite determined. "What's a friend for?" he said. "He helped us when we were having a hard time. He's going through a difficult time now."

The once-thriving industrial city was flattened to the ground. By the time Wende got to Tangshan, there were still numerous people trapped under buildings, dead or alive. At first, the rescuers used their bare hands, but soon after utilized shovels and bulldozers. The whole city reeked with the strong odor of dead bodies. The water was undrinkable.

Wende's old friend kept the body of his daughter in a tent for three days until it began to smell. He was consumed by grief. After the quake, he and his wife managed to pull themselves out, but when they dug their daughter out, she was already dead. Out of his three daughters, she was the prettiest one.

Many years ago, I used to comment on how beautiful she was. "If you like her, I'll marry her to your son Xianping," he said jokingly to me. Wende stayed with his old friend for three days.

After the Tangshan earthquake, we were ordered to move out of apartments and live temporarily in tents just in case of an earthquake. Our family lived in a leaky tent for more than forty days during the rainy autumn. There was a sense of panic in the air, and the land was rife with gossip due to the lack of official closure. Shortly before the earthquake, some people reported catching sight of multicolored lights glittering in the dark sky, while others witnessed fireballs dashing across the sky over their heads, accompanied by an extremely loud sound like roaring thunder. Those stories left such horrifying images inside people.

Old folks considered the quake as an omen, a sign of unknown change. Rumors of Chairman Mao's imminent death began to circulate within days of the quake, even though the media continued to say he was healthy. The chairman had not been seen in public for months, and this was an unmistakable sign in politics that something was wrong. A few months later, it turned out that the "grapevine news" was right. Somehow, in those days, gossip held more truth than the official news.

On September 9, 1976, just when we were about to take off the black armbands we wore in tribute to Premier Zhou and Marshal Zhu, who had passed away at the beginning of the year, Chairman Mao died. That whole year, we mourned the death of important leaders by wearing the black armbands. Mourning music was heard on the loudspeakers every day. Many people fainted during the long memorial service. Entertainment of any kind was forbidden. The only movies we were allowed to watch were documentaries about the funerals of Premier Zhou, Marshal Zhu, and Chairman Mao.

Half a million people attended the chairman's massive funeral in Tiananmen Square. Hua Guofeng, Mao's successor, delivered a memorial speech. He later became known for the

Two Whatevers proposition: whatever Chairman Mao said was right, and whatever Chairman Mao did was right. Shortly afterward, every household respectfully put up Chairman Hua's portrait beside Chairman Mao's. That same year, following Chairman Hua's instruction, Chairman Mao's memorial hall was under construction on the southern side of Tiananmen Square. Even as the nation mourned, power struggles within the party had reached a dramatic stage.

About a month after Chairman Mao's death, the "Gang of Four" — Mao's wife Jiang Qing, together with the other three radicals Zhang Chunqiao, Yao Wenyuan, and Wang Hongwen — were arrested and eventually put on trial in the fall of 1980. Jiang Qing was sentenced to life imprisonment, released for medical reasons in 1991; she committed suicide shortly afterward by hanging herself in the bathroom of her hospital.

All four of Mao's wives suffered a tragic fate. His first wife (arranged marriage) died a year after they married. He abandoned his second wife Yang Kaihui and their children. He drove his third wife, He Zizhen, to madness. Mao ignored his fourth, Jiang Qing, in the later stages of their marriage in favor of pretty young women.

Kang Sheng, the most feared butcher, was accused along with the Gang of Four of being responsible for millions of deaths during the Cultural Revolution, although he had already died of cancer in late 1975. Rumor had it that he was very scared before death came to him. He needed company at all times — day and night, with movies showing constantly.

It took two weeks for the official media to announce the arrest of the Gang of Four. All the crimes that had been committed during the Cultural Revolution were blamed on them. Our old comrades and colleagues finally felt free to contact us after so many years. "It was all caused by the Gang of Four," they said.

The Great Cultural Revolution that had a profound impact on the lives of people and deeply affected the nation's psyche was officially over. It was also the end of Mao's era. According to various sources, during the violent political campaigns from 1950 to 1976, Mao was responsible for as many as 50 million to 80 million deaths. His two famous quotes still linger in the minds of the Chinese people. One was, "A revolution is an uprising, an act of violence whereby one class overthrows another," and the other was, "Political power grows out of the barrel of a gun."

In July 1977, after decades of dramatic political roller-coaster rides, Deng Xiaoping returned to power for the third time and eventually became the paramount leader. On August 12, 1978, China and Japan signed a treaty of peace and friendship, formally normalizing their relationship. In October, Deng made a successful trip to Japan and was impressed by the modern industrial country. He brought back two Japanese movies. One was about a police officer who was framed by his enemy but eventually proved himself innocent. The movie's political implications were apparent, considering that Deng himself had been persecuted three times in the past and eventually had been vindicated; the other movie, a story about a prostitute, caused a huge controversy over its nudity, even though the movie had already been heavily censored by the authorities. For the Chinese people, these two movies were a real eye-opener after being isolated from the rest of the world for almost thirty years. For many years, the only thing people could watch were propaganda movies and a handful of "revolutionary modern model operas," which had been produced by Mao's leftist wife Jiang Qing.

On January 1, 1979, China and the United States established diplomatic relations and shortly after Deng met President Jimmy Carter in the U.S.

The Third Plenum of the Eleventh National Party Congress Central Committee in December 1978 is considered a major turning point in modern Chinese political history. Hua Guofeng's Two Whatevers policy was abolished. It marked the official end of the protracted class struggle, and the beginning of the Four Modernizations in the fields of agriculture, industry, national defense, and science. Deng promptly launched political, economic, social, and cultural reforms. Unlike Chairman Mao, who had persisted with the socialist ideology, he believed that "it doesn't matter if the cat is black or white; it is a good cat as long as it catches mice." This was in direct contrast to the slogan "better red than expert" of Mao's era. Deng was aware that the key to his success lay with the peasants, the majority of the population. After the Great Leap Forward and the People's Commune disaster, Deng had given each peasant a small plot for private use and allowed peasants to operate small sideline businesses. Now he reintroduced the policy after the disruption of the Cultural Revolution, and it produced great initial success. He encouraged peasants to become rich. If Mao were alive, he would definitely accuse Deng of restoring capitalism.

During this period of time, Wende became very excited over the new developments, even though they were not directly related to him. That was all he talked about — although he had some reservations when he heard that women in Beijing started using lipstick, which was considered to be a part of the bourgeois lifestyle just a year earlier. "Is that necessary?" he said. This was a period of such rapid change that people could hardly keep up.

Another dramatic policy reversal from Mao's era was the one concerning birth control. Mao had believed in "more people, more power." His belief was reflected in his "human sea strategy," which was utilized in the disastrous mass movement of the Great Leap Forward when he mobilized the population of the entire country to overtake the capitalist nations. The population had nearly doubled — from 540 million in 1949 to 1 billion by the late 1970s — despite the millions who perished from starvation during the early 1960s. During Mao's time, I often heard the expression "China is a vast country with a large population and abundant resources." However, this is far from reality. China makes up one-quarter of mankind but only has seven percent of the world's arable land, which is dwindling due to decades of environmental destruction.

Now more people, more burden. "One-child policy" was issued after Deng became the paramount leader. Extreme measures such as forced abortion, forced sterilization, and stiff financial penalties were taken in an attempt to control the population. Even though I didn't work in the Gynecology Department, I saw many women come to the hospital in various stages of pregnancy to have abortions. It was easier for the doctors to handle when they were just two or three months' pregnant, but if they were already seven or eight months, the doctors had to induce labor, which tends to be more intense and painful for the women. In these cases, the infants would often come out crying. After the procedure doctors would usually instruct nurses to apply bandages over the infants' mouth until they suffocated. Some women would escape to live with their relatives far away to avoid abortion.

My neighbor Liu, a nurse, became a victim of the unpopular policy. She and her husband already had a three-year-old daughter, but they wanted a boy. It's the traditional preference in Chinese families, especially in the countryside, where producing girls was considered dishonorable. Adhering to One-child policy resulted in frequent female infanticides by parents who wanted boys, sex-selective abortion, and imbalanced male-female birth ratios. Female infanticides were most common during the Qing Dynasty and again since the time when one child policy was enforced.

In the beginning stage of Liu's pregnancy, the hospital leaders urged her to have an abortion. She was very hesitant; her husband was determined to have the baby. When her pregnancy reached eight months, the hospital officials stepped up their pressure on her. Her husband, who had a bad temper, was outraged, and threatened the hospital leaders' lives. He was immediately arrested. While he was in custody, Liu was forced to have an induced labor. She was a very timid person and eventually yielded to the intense pressure. She described to me later that during the procedure she could hear her baby's cries. Her husband remains unforgiving of Deng Xiaoping. He was loyal to Mao, even though his grandmother starved to death during the famine in the early 1960s.

The Cultural Revolution ended in 1976. In the same year, Yanping graduated from high school. She had started school in 1966 when the Cultural Revolution began. She didn't get to learn much in school during those days. Even though our family had just come back from the countryside, she had to return, since all of the educated youth in the towns and cities were being sent to the countryside to do manual labor. This mass movement started at the end of 1968 when Mao issued a directive stating that "educated young people should go to the countryside to be re-educated by poor and lower-middle class peasants."

In the fall, I went to the bus station to see Yanping off. Many parents accompanied their children for the same reason. The band was playing, and slogans were posted on the bus. An official gave a speech, saying it was "glorious to go to the countryside." I said goodbye as Yanping boarded the bus bound for a fishing village in the Shandong Peninsula. No one had any idea how long they would be in the countryside. It turned out that this was the last wave of "educated young people going to the countryside." Just a few months later, the policy was abolished.

In October, I went to the fishing village to visit my daughter. I had assumed that the life was very hard there. To my surprise, she looked quite healthy. She had even gained some weight doing manual labor and eating a lot of fresh seafood. When I came home and told Wende about it, he was relieved.

In September 1978, I started to experience an irregular heart-beat along with pain. Accompanied by Wende, I went to see a doctor at the Qingdao Academy of Medical Sciences. The head of the Cardiovascular System Department diagnosed me as having heart disease caused by viral infection. The method of treatment was to take vitamins, such as B12, for one month. After one month, there was no improvement at all. In October, I went back to the same hospital, this time seeing a different doctor. He looked at my record, and kept shaking his head when he saw the signature belonging to the head of the department. It turned out that the doctor didn't agree with his superior's diagnosis, but he didn't dare to change it because he was a "rightist" working under supervision.

"Continue the treatment for another month and come back for a follow-up," the doctor said.

I thought it was really ridiculous. If it didn't work, why continue for another month? So I went to the Taixi Hospital, another major hospital in the city. A doctor diagnosed my heart disease as caused by rheumatism, not viral infection. The method of treatment was injection of antibiotics and also aspirin to treat the rheumatoid arthritis in my knee that I'd developed during the Korean War. After only two weeks, I felt much better.

Just a few months later, all the intellectuals who had been branded as "rightists" during the Anti-Rightist movement in 1957 were gradually rehabilitated. It was about a year and a half after Deng Xiaoping had been returned to power. Due to the hard labor and the nation-wide famine soon after the Anti-Rightist campaign, many of them had perished. During the Great Cultural Revolution that followed a few years later, the rightists were under attack again. Therefore, when the rehabilitation finally came in 1978 — twenty years later — it was said that out of over half a million rightists in 1957, there were only a little over a hundred thousand survivors.

During that time, I was sent to the Jiaonan County Hospital, where I had worked before, to take a two-month course in traditional Chinese medicine. The government was promoting the policy of combining traditional Chinese medicine and Western medicine. This generally meant using herbs and Western medicine at the same time, and combining the old diagnostic method of feeling the pulse with the use of modern laboratory tests. Often Western medicine was literarily "combined" with the Chinese herbs. I met up with Dr. Chen. The last time I had seen him was when he was escorted by the Red Guard to the countryside. He was doing quite well.

Dr. Chen's reputation had been restored. In the old days they said: "The more knowledge you have, the more reactionary you are." But now they said: "Knowledge is power," which meant that intellectuals were now considered very important. The village chief in Wende's hometown was right when he said, "The policies of the Communist Party can change at any time."

Dr. Chen gloriously became a member of the Communist Party and the leader of the Operating Department. From what I knew, Dr. Chen's children still called him "Uncle." It was hard to change the habit after so many years. Dr. Chen didn't seem to be too concerned about it. We talked just a few minutes. He was very busy and not approachable like he had been before. Did he still remember the food ration I had lent him during the early sixties? I wondered.

In 1979, at the age of fifteen, Luping started high school. Wende rode his bike for hours to another town in order to buy a phonograph for his son to study English. He also wrote to his fellow-villager who lived in Beijing and asked him to send some English course records. As Luping started to repeat the foreign words he heard on the phonograph, Wende listened with pride, though he didn't understand a word. The study of English became very popular after Deng Xiaoping became the paramount leader and opened the door to the rest of the world.

It was at that point that Wende developed the idea of writing a memoir. On several occasions he spoke of his ambitious plan. "This is our history," he said. However, he hesitated. "But what if there is another political movement? It will be evidence that they can use against me. Black words on white paper." He never wrote a word. His memoir ended up as just a big dream that never materialized.

Wende had two favorite books. One was *From Emperor to Citizen*, an autobiography of the last emperor, Pu Yi, who collaborated with the Japanese by becoming the head of Manchuria, and was eventually reformed by the Communists. Another book was the Chinese classic novel *A Dream of the Red Mansions*, a tragic story about the fall of a powerful aristocratic family.

Near the end of 1979, Wende fell ill with liver disease. The stress over the years due to his persecution had taken a heavy toll on his health. In fact, he had suffered from chronic depression ever since his persecution in 1970. A doctor of traditional Chinese medicine took Wende's pulse and prescribed some herbal medicine for him to take. He told Wende that he should try to ease his mind and not to worry so much all the time because "chronic depression hurts the liver."

The medicine contained many kinds of herbs. I placed all the herbs and several cups of water into an earthenware pot, covered it tightly, and then boiled it over a low flame for a long time — until nearly half of the liquid had evaporated. After simmering the mixture for several hours, I strained it through cheesecloth and divided the decoction into two portions for Wende to take in the morning and evening on an empty stomach. He hated the thick, dark brown liquid.

"Bitter medicine cures sickness," I said to him. One course of treatment was ten days. There were a few days between each course. The full course lasted for six months without showing any effect.

Wende's illness coincided with some dramatic changes in the family. During those years, all the children were leaving home. Xianping married in 1980, and moved to Jinan. About two years later, Yanping married, and transferred to Jinan where her husband works. Luping went to high school in Jiaonan First High School, only coming home every six months. We were facing an empty nest.

In September 1980, I accompanied Wende to the Qingdao Academy of Medical Sciences. He was given an herbal medicine almost identical to the prescription he had taken back at home. He came home from Qingdao and drank the bitter decoction for a full course that lasted another six months.

In August of 1981, I accompanied Wende to Beijing Xiehe Hospital. We stayed with Wende's fellow-villager. As usual, the hospital was crammed with people. It took a whole day for him to get a blood test and an X-ray. Even a healthy person would become sick after going through the long procedure! The herbal medicine he was given was identical to the ones he had taken before.

The next day, after the checkup in the hospital, Wende wanted to go to see Chairman Mao's body at Memorial Hall in Tiananmen Square, even though he wasn't feeling well.

There was a long lineup in front of Chairman Mao's memorial hall. We waited for one hour and thirty minutes in the hot sun before we finally got in. Everyone had to check their bags at the checkroom. The line came in through a door where the left side of Chairman Mao's head was positioned. Chairman Mao lay in his crystal coffin, his face looking bloated. Two armed soldiers were standing beside the coffin. We walked in a line, not allowed to stop and take a close look. It was very quiet and I could only hear the rustling sound of clothes. We hastily moved around under Chairman Mao's feet and made a circle to the right side of his head, then quickly exited through another door. We only caught a passing glance of Chairman Mao. After paying our respects, we left Memorial Hall.

"Remember when I was going to come to Beijing to see Chairman Mao in 1967 but the army didn't want me to come? Well, I didn't get to see Chairman Mao alive, but now I've seen him dead," Wende said.

It wasn't the same, but he still seemed honored and satisfied. It was something he just had to do, probably because his wish to see Chairman Mao had not come true the first time.

In the afternoon, when we got back to the fellow-villager's place, we told the old man that we had gone to Chairman Mao's Memorial Hall. The old man put his hand up to Wende's ear and whispered the current "grapevine news":

"The body is just a wax figure. The real one decomposed a long time ago."

21

Evil Ghost

On a hot evening in early August of 1984, a year after I was transferred to Qihe County Hospital, Wende and I were sitting in the yard to cool off after I came home from work. A big snake slithered into the house and settled behind the water vat. Wende used a pair of tongs to grip the snake, and threw it outside unharmed. My hair would stand on end whenever I saw a snake.

A few evenings later, the same thing happened again. This time the snake coiled around the water vat. It was possible, I thought, that the snake enjoyed the coolness of the water vat. Wende used the pair of tongs to send the uninvited guest out without a scratch.

As we were sitting in the yard in the hot evening a few days later, Wende suddenly got up without saying a word, and looked around for something.

"What are you looking for?" I asked him.

He didn't reply, and continued to look until he found the pair of tongs. That was the third time the snake had crawled into the house. He knew I was afraid of snakes so he didn't mention anything. This time the snake had gone under the bed. He tried a long time but couldn't catch it. When he finally managed to capture the snake, it was not moving, and I couldn't tell if it was dead or alive. An old retired neighbor came for a chat. When we told him what had happened, he said: "You should never have harmed the snake. People in this area worship snakes."

"I didn't want to harm it. I just tried to get it out," Wende said to him.

"It's good luck when a snake comes into your home. I have lived here for many years but rarely see a snake," the old neighbor said.

On August 12, shortly after the incident, Wende fell seriously ill. The day coincided with lunar July 15, the Ghost Festival. He was sent to the hospital at four in the afternoon when the neighbors started to burn "paper money" — paper made to resemble money — as an offering to the dead. If people were near to the grave of their deceased family members, they would go there to hold the memorial ceremonies. However, if they were too far away, they would burn the "paper money" on a crossroads, where all the deities and ghosts were believed to pass through.

"It is an ominous time to get sick," the old neighbor said.

The night before Wende was sent to the hospital, he had a dream. A truckload of uniformed soldiers arrived at the door and dragged him onto the truck without saying anything. He grabbed a brick to fight back. It was the only time in his life that he ever told me about his dreams. "Those bastards!" he kept swearing the next morning. When I spoke of the matter with the old neighbor, he said that the ruler of the underworld had sent his servants to take Wende's soul away.

The children were all called back with telegrams. With everyone in the family reunited, an ill omen hung in the air, since separation seemed more normal for us.

The light was very dim in the hospital ward. The room was permeated with a thick, unpleasant odor of sickness. Just a few days earlier, it had been in that very ward where I, together with a few other doctors, had held group consultations for a patient who was terminally ill, and had witnessed his death. Of course, I didn't tell Wende anything about it. In fact I didn't tell anyone at the time.

That night, I dreamt that someone gave me a pair of shoes. I could see the shoes were bright red. I had rarely seen color so vividly in my dreams. "How could I wear such bright red shoes at my age?" I thought to myself in the dream. So I gave my daughter Yanping and Xianping's wife each one of the shoes to wear. Next day, Xianping's wife came to the hospital with my lunch. I felt guilty eating in the ward because Wende was unable to eat anything. He was fed through the tube at the time. I came out of ward, and told my dream to Xianping's wife, who was very straightforward and highly verbal. "The dream is always the opposite. Red is white," she said without thinking. White, of course, was the color of mourning.

Wende became very sentimental as he recalled his past. It seemed that everything made him sad. "I wish we had gotten killed in the Korean War. Then we wouldn't have had to go through those ordeals in our lives," he said.

"You shouldn't be so pessimistic. Things were not as bad as you think," I said to him.

"I heard the cry of owls last night. It's a sign of imminent death according to folklore," he said.

"Try to get better for our children," I said.

"Our children are all grown-up now. Xianping and Yanping are both married. I don't need to worry too much finally. Only one thing — Luping hasn't married yet, and you will have to take care of the matter by yourself now," he said. Even in his last days, he was still worrying about everyone.

Wende's illness became worse. He had a complication and his liver and kidneys had failed. The doctor announced to the family that the patient was critically ill. Several tubes had to be inserted into his nose and mouth. At the same time, he was also being given intravenous medication. A blood transfusion was administered on a daily basis due to his internal bleeding. Wende could no longer speak. He asked for a pen and paper to try to write something. A long time passed, but he didn't write one word. I wondered what he wanted to say.

Since the internal bleeding was impossible to stop, a doctor recommended Yunnan Baiyao, a white herbal powder that could stop bleeding. According to folklore, in ancient times, a farmer in Yunnan found a snake near his hut, and beat it with a hoe, leaving it for dead. A few days later he was surprised to discover the same snake slithering in his yard, and again he tried to kill it. He watched the bleeding snake crawl into a cluster of weeds, and begin eating them. By the next morning, its wounds had healed again. That was how the white powder was discovered.

Luping immediately took a train to Jinan to buy the medicine. As soon as he was away, Wende's condition got worse. The miracle powder didn't save his life.

He died at midnight of September 3, 1984, twenty-one days after his hospitalization. I watched his last struggle, and kept calling his name. At the final moment, he lifted his head, fought for his last breath, then fell back, and expelled the last air from his lungs. "Wende! Wende!" I kept calling. His eyes rolled toward me and froze there for eternity.

Yanping and Luping didn't get to see their father alive for the last time. He died while they were on the way to the hospital. Xianping was the only child beside his father's bed when he passed away.

I sent a telegraph to the 201 Division to inform them about Wende's death, but no one showed up for his funeral. I also sent a telegraph to Wende's relatives. Later I heard that after receiving the telegraph, Guangde had paced up and down in the yard the whole night, crying while his wife was swearing at him in the house. She didn't want him to go to his brother's funeral.

After Wende was cremated, his ash urn was placed in a storage room on a shelf with many others. I promised myself I was going to find him a proper burial place later, but I didn't think it would take me eleven years to do so.

Probably out of paranoia, Xianping decided to burn all the letters and documents his father had accumulated over the years. The fire lasted two hours. Only some of the letters that were locked in my drawer were saved.

When the children were all away, I would wake up in the middle of the night, and turn the light on, searching around the house. I felt a very strong sense of Wende's presence in the house. I had heard that after people died, they could turn into evil spirits, and return after seven days to haunt their homes.

In October, about a month after Wende had passed away, my son Luping and I took his ash urn and went to the 201 Division, which was located in Laiwu, in the south of Shandong Province, to demand a proper burial place for him. Even though it was still the 201 Division, the people were all new. I didn't recognize a single face. A young officer had received me. He waited impatiently for me to finish my story.

"Your husband's burial site is now the responsibility of the local government. There's nothing we can do," he said.

"My husband dedicated his heart and soul to the army for twenty-five years. He died because he was treated unjustly. Now he can't even have a proper burial place."

"You husband died of natural diseases. It has nothing to do with us," he said.

"His illness was caused by the stress during the Cultural Revolution when he was persecuted by the 201 Division. How can you say it has nothing to do with you?" I said.

"What evidence do you have that his illness was caused by us?" he said. "It was caused by the Gang of Four. You have to look forward, put the past behind you," the official said.

I was infuriated by his words. "I'm tired of hearing it's all caused by the Gang of Four. You were all in on it. All of you," I said.

I stayed there for two months without results. In December, Luping and I took Wende's ash urn and went to the General

Political Department in Beijing. It was an extremely cold winter. The day I went to the office, it was snowing heavily, and the streets were very slippery. Several times I was almost fell to the ground. I waited the whole day to see someone in the office. When the interview was over, I almost fainted because I hadn't eaten the whole day. I was told that they couldn't do anything about it, and that I had to go to the 201 Division, who had handled Wende's case directly. I was given the runaround for many years.

AFTERWORD

———

Two YEARS AFTER Wende passed away, I retired from the hospital, and worked part-time in a private clinic in Jinan for a few years with a colleague of mine who was also retired. Striving to carry out Wende's aspiration, I started writing a family memoir. It also gave me something to do when I felt lonely. I was fated to be alone. Remember the fortune-teller said I had the fate of a nun? Anyway, I completed over fifty pages, from the time I was young up until the Cultural Revolution. But in the end, just like Wende, I became afraid of causing trouble, and burned the writing to ashes.

Since Wende passed away, many things have happened in my family. Yanping had a baby girl about two years after her father passed away. She worked in a department store for many years, then was laid off because the government-run store closed. She became a housewife after that and seems content with her life. Luckily her husband has a secure job so they don't need to worry about their living conditions like the millions of unemployed. Like her brother Xianping, she was also deprived of an education during the Cultural Revolution, and left without any usable skills. However, she was never resentful over this fact. Her mild temper reminds me of Wende. She's a very good mother, devoting a lot of time to her child.

Xianping divorced his wife in 1989, citing irreconcilable differences as the reason. I liked her. She was a very enthusiastic and outspoken person. Their divorce procedure took some time to come through, and coincided with the June Fourth movement or Tiananmen Square Massacre, which she attended. Since 1978, Deng had steered a series of economic and political reforms that had led to the gradual accomplishment of a market economy and some political liberalization. Between April 15 and June 4, students, intellectuals, and urban workers began a series of demonstrations centered on Tiananmen Square in Beijing, but soon spread into cities throughout the country. The protesters ranged from intellectuals who believed the Communist Party was too corrupt and repressive, to urban workers who believed the economic reform had gone too far, resulting in runaway inflation and massive unemployment. On the night of June 3 and the early morning of June 4, army tanks and infantry were sent into Tiananmen Square to crush the protest. Several hundred civilians were killed and thousands were injured during the bloody military operation. The government never hesitates to resort to violence. As a veteran, I was shocked at the fact that the army had turned its guns on their own people. Following the violence, the government conducted nationwide arrests of the movement supporters, and tightened its control over the foreign and domestic press. Xianping's ex-wife was reprimanded by the authorities at her workplace, but luckily nothing serious happened to her. She and I remained friends for years after their divorce until she moved to France. In 1991, Luping crossed the Pacific Ocean and started a new life in Canada.

In early April of 1994, during the Qingming festival, the day when people visit the graves of their family members, I went with my daughter Yanping to visit Wende's ash urn at the crematorium. Many such urns were piled up in a storage room and it took me a long time to find his.

"You were treated unjustly when you were alive, and you died without a place for burial," I said to his urn.

I decided to take it home with me.

From the moment his urn came into the house, I began experiencing a constant sore throat and a twitching right eyelid, which was commonly believed to be an omen of disaster. My premonition came true. In July, Luping got into a serious car accident in Canada. In September, I was getting out of a bus, and the driver drove away before my feet landed firmly on the ground. As a result, I hit my head on the ground and fainted. I rested in bed for a week. I didn't tell Luping at the time because I didn't want him to worry. Could Wende have turned into an evil spirit as the folklore said? He was such a harmless person, but could it be possible that he had transformed into a fearful spirit after he died? How could he harm his own family?

"I'm going to throw you out," I shouted at the ash urn angrily. "How could you do harm to me and to our son? I have done my best to find you a burial place. I went to the 201 Division, and I went to the General Political Department in Beijing. What else can I do? I thought you would like it when I brought you back home. And this is how you thank me?"

That night, I dreamt Wende was standing beside my bed with tears in his eyes. "Please don't throw me out. It wasn't my fault," he said.

On September 3, 1995, eleven years to the day that Wende passed away, he finally received a respectful burial. We had bought a burial place on a mountain in the suburbs of Jinan.

The route to the burial site was bumpy and winding. There was a fair going on in one of the villages we were passing by, and the taxi had to zigzag its way through. A picture of Chairman Mao was dangling on the driver's rear-view mirror. Chairman Mao, kind and Buddha-like, was swinging back and forth. The driver told me that with a picture of Chairman Mao in the car, he was protected, and would never get into an accident. Even though Chairman Mao had died many years ago, people still revered him. His status was elevated to that of a deity.

It was drizzling that day. There was some water at the bottom of the pit so I took my scarf off and placed it down to cover the water. We burned "paper money" and incense in front of Wende's tomb as an offering to him. The tomb was built with stone and raised a couple of feet above the ground. In front of it was the black marble tombstone that bore Wende's name engraved in white and mine in red beside his. The names of the children, and the grandchildren whom he'd never met, were on the left side in smaller characters. Clearly marked were the dates Wende was born and died. The tomb was only the first phase of work, so it didn't yet look like what Luping saw in 1997 when he and his wife visited it. A short wall was to be built later at the back of the tomb to prevent mud slides during the rain.

"Like the old saying goes: 'Peace under the earth,'" I said to the children. "I hope your father finally found peace." *Ru tu wei an* — the Chinese believe that a deceased person can only find peace after being buried in the soil.

After the burial, I had several recurring dreams that Wende came to me and complained that the house was leaking due to the rain. This is called *tuo meng*, and refers to an old belief that the ghost of one's kin appears in one's dream to make a request. That was when I found out that the second phase of the work hadn't been completed on his tomb. My recurring dreams didn't stop until they finished the job a few months later. Xianping took a picture of the tomb and sent a copy to Luping in Canada. After the photo was developed, we noticed there was a colorful rainbow across Wende's tombstone. We believed that Wende's spirit had made its presence known, and this was such a comforting feeling.

In the spring of 1996, I finally had a chance to visit Luping and his wife in Regina, Canada. Xianping accompanied me on the train from Jinan to Beijing. At the Beijing International Airport he said to me: "Mom, don't talk about the Korean War when you are in Canada. Canadians were part of the UN force during the war."

"Who am I going to tell?" I said.

We sat in the waiting room at the airport for a long time. "Stay in Canada," Xianping said to me when the boarding started. He waited until my plane took off before leaving airport. At the Immigration Department of the Vancouver airport, I realized that he had only bought me a one-way ticket. The female immigration officer who spoke Mandarin questioned why I only had a one-way ticket while holding a visitor's visa. I couldn't answer the question but eventually they let me pass. Luping and his wife, Patty, came to the airport to meet me. I arrived in Vancouver at just the right time — when all cherry trees along the streets were in full bloom. We stayed in Vancouver for two nights and then took a plane to Regina.

I knew two things about Canada. Dr. Norman Bethune, who went to China to help the Communists against the Japanese, was one of them. Mao had written an essay entitled "In Memory of Norman Bethune," and called people to learn "the spirit of absolute selflessness from him." The other thing was Canadian wheat. Older Chinese still remember that it was Canadian wheat that came to the rescue near the end of the 1960s famine.

Luping's intention was to let me live with them in Canada. However, I couldn't get used to the life there, even though there are many modern conveniences, like private baths and cars. Water is plentiful there, not like in China where people have to be very careful when it comes to water and electricity. Except for cooking meals, there wasn't much for me to do. Since a young age, I was raised to keep busy, active, and independent. But in this strange place, I couldn't go in and out as I pleased; I always had to be accompanied by Luping or Patty. Luping bought me a short-wave radio, hoping that I could receive Chinese programs, but it was very difficult to tune and eventually I gave it up. Luckily, there was a fairly big park right in front of the apartment. So every day I would come out of confinement like a prisoner to have a walk in the park, but I couldn't stray out of the sight of my children.

It was in this park I met up with an elderly Chinese woman. We immediately warmed up to each other. She came to Canada to take care of her grandchild and only occasionally came out to get some fresh air. I looked forward to meeting her in the park. We met several times until one day she failed to show up and I never saw her again. I never found out what happened. Maybe her children didn't want her to talk to strangers.

I told Luping about my intention to go back to China.

"Canada is a beautiful country and we have good living conditions here, so why can't you live here?" he said to me.

"Like the old saying goes, the falling leaves settle on the roots," I said. "China is my roots. I'm used to the life there."

I only stayed for a few months before I headed back to China. During that time, Luping and his wife were planning a move to Vancouver. On the eve of the move, I dreamt Wende came to help with the moving. "I took a leave to help Luping move. I only earn twenty yuan a month. Because I took the leave, they have deducted ten yuan off my pay," he said. Since then, every time my family goes to visit his grave, we always burn the "paper money" as an offering.

As we were driving down the Trans-Canada Highway, I was deeply impressed by the vast wheat fields and tall grain elevators on the prairies, and the majestic Rockies. It took us three days to get to Vancouver by car. I felt blessed to be able to see all those things at my age.

✪

Xianping stayed single for about ten years following his divorce, then remarried in 1998, and had a son the next year. When the boy was born, I had to take buses to the hospital to bring food for his mother. I took very good care of my grandson for a couple of years. It was tiring work, but it certainly brought me a lot of happiness. Traditionally, it was the grandparents' duty to take care of the grandchildren.

At the end of the year 2000, my friend's son, a professional photographer, came to videotape my grandson so I could send a tape to Luping and his wife in Canada. I knew they would be very happy to see it. In the middle of the taping, Luping called me and wanted me to head to Vancouver for a visit. I wanted to go and stay for a few months, but I couldn't leave because Xianping and his wife were both working. As always it was difficult to find a good babysitter. My daughter-in-law had found three young girls from her hometown, but none had worked out. The first one was only fourteen so she missed her family and returned home shortly. The second one had some kind of illness. The third one didn't know how to do anything, and was sensitive to even the slightest criticism. She cried more often than the baby, and quit after two weeks. We didn't want to try the employment agencies because I had heard of cases where children had been abducted by babysitters. Besides, those babysitters were too expensive. I knew how difficult it was to find a trustworthy nanny because I'd had the same experience when I had my own children. If I took care of my grandson for one more year — until he was about three — we could send him to kindergarten, which Xianping could take him to and from. It would be less work and I would be free. I wish that I had been given the chance to spend so much time with my own children when they were young.

My grandson was a handsome little guy. He already knew over forty Chinese characters, all the English letters, and could say "okay." He could pretty much say anything. I often took him outside to play. "My uncle and auntie live in Canada," he always told anyone he met.

One night, when my grandson was about two years old, we were drinking milk at the table.

"Good boy," I said to him. "Drink your milk. Look, Grandma is drinking milk."

"Grandpa drinks milk too," he suddenly said.

I was startled by it. I couldn't help looking around the room. It was strange because no one had ever mentioned anything about Grandpa to him. They say that because children are innocent, they can see things the grown-ups can't. Could that be right?

I have never gotten along with Xianping's second wife since she first came through the door. So I moved out and lived by myself. Xianping wasn't happy about it. Traditionally parents always live with children. It is the sons' duty to take care of aging parents.

"Ma, you are blessed to live with your son and grandson. It's a perfect situation. Why can't you live peacefully with us?" he said to me.

"I have the fate of a nun. I'm meant to be alone," I said.

My daughter Yanping was quite upset upon hearing the news of my moving out. There was an argument between her and Xianping. Luping was thousands of miles away and was frustrated with everyone for quarrelling. I felt sad about the disharmony within the family. Throughout my family history, especially during the Cultural Revolution, our family had always struggled to stay together. Now it seemed that the family was falling apart.

I had been living with Xianping ever since his divorce. I cooked for him and took good care of him. He still has difficulties reconciling with the past. Because of his loss of education and military career, he was resentful of not only the government, but also of Wende and me. As a mother, I understand his feelings. He is the oldest child, and suffered the most during the Cultural Revolution. When Wende was persecuted, I had a difficult decision to make. I could have divorced Wende. Then my children would have been able to stay with me, and would have had a chance for a better education and career. Of course, out of loyalty, I chose to go to the countryside with Wende. It would be dishonest to say I never had any doubts about my decision. In those circumstances, any decision would be a wrong decision.

In the fall of 2001, I visited Luping and his wife for a second time in Canada. It was a beautiful season in Vancouver. The maple trees had turned bright red all over the city. It was just shortly after the terrorist attack of September 11th and there was still a sense of panic in the air. Because of the anthrax scare, the children washed all of my clothes the night I arrived.

With their help, I continued working on this memoir. During the process, Luping and I got into an argument. Something from the past brought out the high emotions from deep inside of us. Luping believed that his father shouldn't have taken herbal medicine for such an extended period of time. Recent studies have shown many of the ingredients are toxic, often causing liver and kidney failure.

Mystical traditional Chinese medicine, an integral part of Chinese philosophy, essentially has not changed over the course of 5,000 years of history. It held its ground in the face of apparent Western medicine miracles introduced to China in the beginning of the century. It has survived despite attempts to ban herbal medicine in the late 1920s by Chinese doctors who studied Western medicine overseas. Even though anything traditional was swept away during the Cultural Revolution, this ancient system was kept intact. Even though Mao had called traditional Chinese medicine a "great treasure-house," his motive was more political than medical. Ironically, the simple fact that his personal physician was Western-trained revealed that he himself didn't trust Chinese medicine. However, Mao knew that he couldn't abandon Chinese medicine — it was his cultural foundation.

I do regret that I had let Wende take herbal medicine for such an extended period of time. Even though I didn't have blind faith in the herbs, it wasn't easy to see the truth behind the fantasy veil. Now I realize that traditional Chinese medicine is just like *mi hun tang* — a deceiving potion according to folklore which spirits are forced to drink in order to forget their previous life before reincarnation. Today, traditional medicine is still an integral part of China's health-care system. It continues to deceive most of the Chinese people, especially the ignorant peasants. The most deceptive government policy is "combining traditional Chinese medicine with Western medicine," a philosophy that resembled Jesus's Chinese brother Hong Xiuquan's strange formulation of pre-Confucian utopianism with Protestant beliefs. It's almost like the obsolete herbal medicine is trying to *jie shi huan hun* where a dead person's soul finds reincarnation in another's corpse and something evil is revived in a new guise. No wonder Lu Xun said that "traditional Chinese medicine doctors are intentionally or unintentionally deceiving their patients." The famous writer Lu Xun (1881–1936) blamed herbal medicine for his father's death. He wrote in an essay that to cure his father's illness, an herbalist sent the child Lu Xun to search for an important ingredient — a pair of crickets that had to be in their first marriage.

Luping also questioned why I didn't seek out treatment earlier for his deceased second brother Bingbing. As a doctor, I blamed myself for not being able to save my own husband and son, not to mention many other people. Luping was also resentful that I never spent much time with them as they were growing up, especially during the Cultural Revolution when we were split up into three parts. Xianping had the same opinion. "Where were you when we needed a mother?" he said to me once. I wish they could understand the circumstances at the time. Nevertheless, I'm proud of the fact that Luping values our family history so much.

"I finally understand why my father often described the Cultural Revolution as an event that had 'touched people to their innermost soul,'" Luping said to me after the memoir was complete.

The second time I stayed in Vancouver for five months, celebrated my birthday, and later Christmas for the first time in my life. However, my arthritis became worse because of the rainy winters in Vancouver. I left the country in mid-March of 2002. Luping and Patty came to the airport to see me off. The plane took off in the early afternoon and landed in Beijing the next day around four o'clock in the afternoon, local time. My daughter Yanping was waiting for me at the gate. She bought us train tickets for ten that night to Jinan. Since the train station was as crowded as usual, we decided to wait a couple of hours at the airport before we headed out on a bus. It was an hour bus ride to the train station and we waited there for a long time before boarding. Even though we had sleepers — small bunks — I couldn't sleep at all. So we chatted. It was four o'clock in the morning when we arrived in Jinan. Yanping didn't go back to her home, but stayed with me at my apartment for the night. I still couldn't sleep.

The next morning, Xianping, his wife, and son came to see me with fresh flowers and a watermelon. My daughter-in-law hugged me and cried. I realized that she'd had a change of heart. During my absence, every so often my grandson would say, "I miss Grandma." In the afternoon, my son-in-law and Yanping's daughter also came with well known Nanjing Salted Duck that he brought back from a business trip. Yanping and I prepared supper. We ate around the table and talked. In great detail, I told them about my experiences in Vancouver. They all left at about nine o'clock in the evening. I was all alone and couldn't sleep. I watched Beijing opera on TV until two in the morning. It might have been jet lag, but I got over it very quickly. Three days later I felt much better and my sleep returned to normal.

I am eighty-one years old now and still planning to appeal. "One of these days, I'll take all your father's writings to the central government. Your father died of injustice," I often tell my children. Most of Wende's documents were burned by Xianping after Wende passed away. I kept some important ones in my drawer. Those documents include appeal letters he wrote to the army after his persecution.

Last winter, I dreamt of Wende. On an extremely hot day, Wende and I met on the opposite side of a highway. I was on the north side and he was on the south side. He was so warm that he took off his army uniform, placing it over his right arm. It was simple and quick, but a very vivid dream.

"Is it true that when people die of injustice they turn into evil ghosts?" I asked.

"The traffic is so busy. Don't cross over," he said to me in his usual slow tone.

About the Authors

Dr. Li Qunying was born in 1926 in Chifeng, Inner Mongolia, China. She joined the Communist army in 1945, and became a medic during the Civil War and the Korean War. After leaving the army, she worked as a doctor in various hospitals throughout Shandong Province for many years. After her husband Han Wende was persecuted in 1970 during the Cultural Revolution, she followed him to the countryside where she became a barefoot doctor. She spent many years seeking justice for her husband, even after his death. She retired as a full-time doctor in 1986, and began working part-time at a private clinic. She now lives an active and independent life in Jinan, Shandong Province, near her children.

———

Louis Luping Han is the youngest son of Dr. Li Qunying. He was born in Shandong Province, China, and grew up during the traumatic Cultural Revolution. He now lives in Vancouver, Canada, with his wife Patty. He encouraged his mother to recall her past, and spent over seven years compiling her memoir.

ACKNOWLEDGEMENTS

We're grateful to our publisher Jack David who believes in this memoir and has worked with us closely in every step of the process. Special thanks to our editor Emily Schultz who did so much to enhance the text, and whose insightful queries led to great improvements. We would also like to thank Dr. Patricia Anderson for her valuable advice. Thanks to everyone in our family for their support. Han Xianping (Louis' brother) contributed a part of the family history from the winter of 1968 to the summer of 1970. Patty (Louis' wife) has spent over seven years in assisting with the work, and shared our emotions and frustration.